Sleep Information for Teens

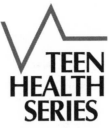

TEEN HEALTH SERIES

First Edition

Sleep Information for Teens

Health Tips about Adolescent Sleep Requirements, Sleep Disorders, and the Effects of Sleep Deprivation

Including Facts about Why People Need Sleep, Sleep Patterns, Circadian Rhythms, Dreaming, Insomnia, Sleep Apnea, Narcolepsy, and More

◆

Edited by Karen Bellenir

Omnigraphics

P.O. Box 31-1640, Detroit, MI 48231

Bibliographic Note
Because this page cannot legibly accommodate all the copyright notices, the Bibliographic Note portion of the Preface constitutes an extension of the copyright notice.

Edited by Karen Bellenir

Teen Health Series
Karen Bellenir, *Managing Editor*
David A. Cooke, M.D., *Medical Consultant*
Elizabeth Collins, *Research and Permissions Coordinator*
Cherry Stockdale, *Permissions Assistant*
EdIndex, Services for Publishers, *Indexers*

* * *

Omnigraphics, Inc.
Matthew P. Barbour, *Senior Vice President*
Kay Gill, *Vice President—Directories*
Kevin M. Hayes, *Operations Manager*

* * *

Peter E. Ruffner, *Publisher*

Copyright © 2008 Omnigraphics, Inc.

ISBN 978-0-7808-1009-9

Library of Congress Cataloging-in-Publication Data

Sleep information for teens / edited by Karen Bellenir.
   p. cm. -- (Teen health series)
   "Health tips about adolescent sleep requirements, sleep disorders, and the effects of sleep deprivation including facts about why people need sleep, sleep patterns, circadian rhythms, dreaming, insomnia, sleep apnea, narcolepsy, and more."
   Includes bibliographical references and index.
   ISBN 978-0-7808-1009-9 (hardcover : alk. paper) 1. Sleep--Handbooks, manuals, etc. 2. Teenagers--Sleep--Handbooks, manuals, etc. 3. Sleep disorders--Handbooks, manuals, etc. I. Bellenir, Karen.
   RA786b.S64 2008
   613.7'940835--dc22

                                                    2007043695

This book is printed on acid-free paper meeting the ANSI Z39.48 Standard. The infinity symbol that appears above indicates that the paper in this book meets that standard.

Printed in the United States

Table of Contents

Part Three: Sleep Disorders And Related Problems

Part Four: The Consequences Of Sleep Deprivation

Part Five: Sleep Research

Part Six: If You Need More Information

Preface

About This Book

A poster produced by the National Heart, Lung, and Blood Institute's "Awake at the Wheel" campaign asks, "Why can't Johnny stay awake in class?" The answer is straightforward: "Because, like other teenagers, he needs at least 9 hours of sleep per night, and he's only getting 6."

Sleep cycles are regulated by an internal biological clock, and when children enter the teen years, their sleep patterns change. They feel more wakeful later into the evening than they did when they were younger. When this natural tendency is coupled with earlier school starting times, sleep debts begin to accumulate. Inadequate sleep leads to poorer daytime performance and a decreased ability to concentrate. It has a negative impact on learning, extracurricular activities, and social relationships. It increases reaction times, contributes to memory lapses, and can affect behavior and moods. When teens don't get enough sleep at night, they fall asleep at inappropriate—and even dangerous—times, such as in class or behind the wheel.

Sleep Information For Teens provides facts about sleep and sleep requirements for teens. It explains the biological processes involved in sleep and discusses circadian rhythms, dreaming, sleep hygiene, and sleep disorders, including insomnia, delayed sleep phase syndrome, sleep apnea, narcolepsy, restless legs syndrome, sleep walking, and enuresis (bedwetting). A special section on sleep deprivation explains the physical and mental consequences of inadequate sleep, and a section on current research initiatives reports some of the most recent findings. The book concludes with a directory of resources for additional information and a list of suggestions for further reading about sleep and sleep disorders.

How To Use This Book

This book is divided into parts and chapters. Parts focus on broad areas of interest; chapters are devoted to single topics within a part.

Part One: Understanding Sleep describes what happens during sleep and why it is so important to health. It discusses the role circadian rhythms play in sleep regulation and talks about the benefits and potential problems related to napping. The part concludes with a look into the mysterious process of dreaming.

Part Two: Sleep Habits examines circumstances and practices that influence the quantity and quality of sleep. It explains how much sleep is needed and offers suggestions for getting sufficient, restful sleep. The effects of caffeine, anxiety, and post-traumatic stress on the ability to sleep are described, and the benefits and risks of sleeping medications and other therapies for sleep problems are discussed.

Part Three: Sleep Disorders And Related Problems provides information about the symptoms, diagnostic procedures, and treatments for common sleep-related disorders, including insomnia, delayed sleep phase syndrome, sleep apnea, and narcolepsy. It also explains such sleep-related behaviors as sleep-walking, nocturnal sleep-related eating disorders, enuresis (bedwetting), and bruxism (teeth grinding). The part concludes with a discussion of lung function changes during sleep that can exacerbate asthma symptoms.

Part Four: The Consequences Of Sleep Deprivation discusses the mental and physical effects of insufficient sleep and explains how a lack of sleep can impact daily functioning. It describes how sleep deprivation can lead to diminished learning and thinking skills, difficulties in handling emotions, and poor physical performance. It also discusses the role sleep deprivation plays in placing teens at increased risk for weight gain and accidents.

Part Five: Sleep Research provides statistical information and summarizes recent discoveries made by investigators who study sleep-related neurological and biological processes. It also provides information about current research initiatives that are underway through several agencies of the National Institutes of Health.

Part Six: If You Need More Information offers a directory of sleep-related resources and suggestions for further reading about sleep and sleep disorders.

Bibliographic Note

This volume contains documents and excerpts from publications issued by the following government agencies: Agency for Healthcare Research and Quality; Body And Mind (BAM!), Centers for Disease Control and Prevention; National Center for Complementary and Alternative Medicine; National Center for Posttraumatic Stress Disorder, Department of Veterans Affairs; National Center on Sleep Disorders Research; National Heart, Lung, and Blood Institute; National Institute of Mental Health; National Institute of Neurological Disorders and Stroke; and the Office of Dietary Supplements.

In addition, this volume contains copyrighted documents and articles produced by the following organizations and individuals: AAA Foundation for Traffic Safety; American Insomnia Association; American Psychiatric Association; American Psychological Association; Anorexia Nervosa and Related Eating Disorders, Inc.; BSCS; Helpguide.org; International Association for the Study of Dreams; Dr. Murray W. Johns; Kidzzzsleep; National Sleep Foundation; Nebraska Rural Health and Safety Coalition, University of Nebraska Medical Center; Nemours Foundation; Oregon State University Student Health Services; and the University of Chicago Medical Center.

Full citation information is provided on the first page of each chapter. Every effort has been made to secure all necessary rights to reprint the copyrighted material. If any omissions have been made, please contact Omnigraphics to make corrections for future editions.

The photograph on the front cover is from Ana Blazic/Shutterstock.

Acknowledgements

In addition to the organizations listed above, special thanks are due to Liz Collins, Research and Permissions Coordinator; Cherry Stockdale, Permissions Assistant; and Elizabeth Bellenir and Nicole Salerno, editorial assistants.

About the *Teen Health Series*

At the request of librarians serving today's young adults, the *Teen Health Series* was developed as a specially focused set of volumes within Omnigraphics' *Health Reference Series*. Each volume deals comprehensively with a topic selected according to the needs and interests of people in middle school and high school.

Teens seeking preventive guidance, information about disease warning signs, medical statistics, and risk factors for health problems will find answers to their questions in the *Teen Health Series*. The *Series*, however, is not intended to serve as a tool for diagnosing illness, in prescribing treatments, or as a substitute for the physician/patient relationship. All people concerned about medical symptoms or the possibility of disease are encouraged to seek professional care from an appropriate health care provider.

If there is a topic you would like to see addressed in a future volume of the *Teen Health Series*, please write to:

Editor
Teen Health Series
Omnigraphics, Inc.
P.O. Box 31-1640
Detroit, MI 48231

Locating Information within the *Teen Health Series*

The *Teen Health Series* contains a wealth of information about a wide variety of medical topics. As the *Series* continues to grow in size and scope, locating the precise information needed by a specific student may become more challenging. To address this concern, information about books within the *Teen Health Series* is included in *A Contents Guide to the Health Reference Series*. The *Contents Guide* presents an extensive list of more than 13,000 diseases, treatments, and other topics of general interest compiled from the Tables of Contents and major index headings from the books of the *Teen Health Series* and *Health Reference Series*. To access *A Contents Guide to the Health Reference Series*, visit www.healthreferenceseries.com.

Our Advisory Board

We would like to thank the following advisory board members for providing guidance to the development of this *Series*:

Dr. Lynda Baker, Associate Professor of Library and Information Science, Wayne State University, Detroit, MI

Nancy Bulgarelli, William Beaumont Hospital Library, Royal Oak, MI

Karen Imarisio, Bloomfield Township Public Library, Bloomfield Township, MI

Karen Morgan, Mardigian Library, University of Michigan-Dearborn, Dearborn, MI

Rosemary Orlando, St. Clair Shores Public Library, St. Clair Shores, MI

Medical Consultant

Medical consultation services are provided to the *Teen Health Series* editors by David A. Cooke, M.D. Dr. Cooke is a graduate of Brandeis University, and he received his M.D. degree from the University of Michigan. He completed residency training at the University of Wisconsin Hospital and Clinics. He is board-certified in internal medicine. Dr. Cooke currently works as part of the University of Michigan Health System and practices in Ann Arbor, MI. In his free time, he enjoys writing, science fiction, and spending time with his family.

Part One

Understanding Sleep

Chapter 1

Facts And Misperceptions About Sleep

Sleep is a behavioral state that is a natural part of every individual's life. We spend about one-third of our lives asleep. Nonetheless, people generally know little about the importance of this essential activity. Sleep is not just something to fill time when a person is inactive. Sleep is a required activity, not an option. Even though the precise functions of sleep remain a mystery, sleep is important for normal motor and cognitive function. We all recognize and feel the need to sleep. After sleeping, we recognize changes that have occurred, as we feel rested and more alert. Sleep actually appears to be required for survival. Rats deprived of sleep will die within two to three weeks, a time frame similar to death due to starvation.[1]

It is not normal for a person to be sleepy at times when he or she expects to be awake. Problem sleepiness may be associated with difficulty concentrating, memory lapses, loss of energy, fatigue, lethargy, and emotional instability. The prevalence of problem sleepiness is high and has serious consequences, such as drowsy driving or workplace accidents and errors. Lifestyle factors and undiagnosed or untreated sleep disorders can cause problem sleepiness. Lifestyle factors include not getting enough sleep, having an irregular sleep schedule, and using alcohol or certain medications. Of the more than 70 known sleep disorders, the most common are obstructive sleep apnea, insomnia, narcolepsy, and restless legs syndrome. Large numbers of individuals suffering from these sleep disorders are unaware of—and have not been diagnosed or treated for—their disorder.[2]

Problem sleepiness can be deadly. Approximately 100,000 automobile crashes each year result from drivers who were "asleep at the wheel." In a survey of drivers in New York State, approximately 25 percent reported they had fallen asleep at the wheel at some time.[3] Crashes in which the driver falls asleep are especially common among young male drivers. One large study found that in over 50 percent of fall-asleep crashes, the driver was 25 years old or younger.[4] In addition to the high risk of automobile crashes, problem sleepiness can cause difficulties with learning, memory, thinking, and feelings, which may lead to poor school and work performance and difficulty with relationships. Further-more, problem sleepiness leads to errors and accidents in the workplace.

Very few textbooks for high school students provide any scientific infor-mation about changes that occur in the body during sleep and how those changes affect our ability to move and think. Of course, we've heard that a good night's sleep will help us perform better on a test the next day, but is this based on scientific fact, or is it just a continuing myth? The lack of information in textbooks may be due to the fact that sleep research is only

✎ What's It Mean?

Insomnia: Sleeplessness; chronic difficulty with sleep onset or maintenance of sleep, or a perception of nonrefreshing sleep.

Narcolepsy: A chronic sleep disorder characterized by excessive and over-whelming daytime sleepiness (even after adequate nighttime sleep).

Obstructive Sleep Apnea (OSA): A disorder in which breathing is frequently interrupted for brief intervals during sleep, resulting in intermittent decreases in blood oxygen levels and transient arousals from sleep, leading to poor sleep quality and excessive daytime sleepiness.

Restless Legs Syndrome: A neuralgic movement disorder that is often asso-ciated with a sleep complaint.

Source: Copyright © 2003 by BSCS.

recently gaining recognition. A great deal remains to be learned through scientific studies, including an answer to the key question, What is the function of sleep? Although its function remains unclear, research is providing a great deal of information about what happens in the brain and body during sleep and how the body regulates sleep.

Misconceptions About Sleep

Students may have misconceptions about what causes us to sleep, what occurs during sleep, how our body responds to a lack of sleep, and what function(s) sleep fulfills. The information in this chapter should help correct the following misconceptions.

Misconception 1: Sleep is time for the body in general and the brain specifically to shut down for rest.

Sleep is an active process involving specific cues for its regulation. Although there are some modest decreases in metabolic rate, there is no evidence that any major organ or regulatory system in the body shuts down during sleep.[1] Some brain activity, including delta waves, increases dramatically. Also, the endocrine system increases secretion of certain hormones during sleep, such as growth hormone and prolactin. In REM sleep, many parts of the brain are as active as at any time when awake.

Misconception 2: Getting just one hour less sleep per night than needed will not have any effect on daytime functioning.

When daily sleep time is less than an individual needs, a "sleep debt" develops. Even relatively modest daily reductions in sleep time (for example, one hour) can accumulate across days to cause a sleep debt. If the debt becomes too great, it can lead to problem sleepiness. Although the individual may not realize his or her sleepiness, the sleep debt can have powerful effects on daytime performance, thinking, and mood.

Misconception 3: The body adjusts quickly to different sleep schedules.

The biological clock that times and controls a person's sleep/wake cycle will attempt to function according to a normal day/night schedule even when

---

♣ **It's A Fact!!**

Why do I need to sleep?

Every creature needs to rest. Giraffes, little babies, elephants, dogs, cats, kids, koala bears, grandparents, moms, dads, and hippos in the jungle—they all sleep. Just like eating, sleep is necessary for survival.

Sleep gives your body a rest and allows it to prepare for the next day. It's like giving your body a mini-vacation. Sleep also gives your brain a chance to sort things out. Scientists aren't exactly sure what kinds of organizing your brain does while you sleep, but they think that sleep may be the time when the brain sorts and stores information, replaces chemicals, and solves problems.

The amount of sleep a person needs depends a lot on his or her age. Babies sleep a lot—about 14 to 15 hours a day! But many older people only need about seven or eight hours of sleep each night. Most kids between the ages of 5 and 12 years old are somewhere in between, needing 10 to 11 hours of sleep. Some kids might need more and some need less. It depends on the kid.

Skipping one night's sleep makes a person cranky and clumsy. After missing two nights of sleep, a person will have problems thinking and doing things; his or her brain and body can't do their normal tasks nearly as well. After five nights without sleep, a person will hallucinate (this means seeing things that aren't actually there). Eventually, it becomes impossible for the brain to give its directions to the rest of the body without sleep—the brain needs to spend time in bed and catch its ZZZs!

Source: This information was provided by KidsHealth, one of the largest resources online for medically reviewed health information written for parents, kids, and teens. For more articles like this one, visit www.KidsHealth.org, or www.TeensHealth.org. © 2007 The Nemours Foundation.

that person tries to change it. Those who work night shifts naturally feel sleepy when nighttime comes. A similar feeling that occurs during travel is known as jet lag. This conflict, set up by trying to be active during the brain's biological nighttime, leads to a decrease in cognitive and motor skills. The biological clock can be reset, but only by appropriately timed cues and even then, by one to two hours per day at best.[5] Problems resulting from a mismatch of this type may be reduced by behaviors such as sleeping in a dark, quiet room, getting exposure to bright light at the right time, and altering eating and exercise patterns. Because humans function best when they sleep at night and act in the daytime, the task for a person who must be active at night is to retrain the biological clock (by light cues).

Misconception 4: People need less sleep as they grow older.

Older people don't need less sleep, but they often get less sleep. That's because the ability to sleep for long periods of time and to get into the deep, restful stages of sleep decreases with age. Many older people have more fragile sleep and are more easily disturbed by light, noise, and pain than when younger. They are also more likely to have medical conditions that contribute to sleep problems.

Misconception 5: A "good night's sleep" can cure problems with excessive daytime sleepiness.

Excessive daytime sleepiness can be associated with a sleep disorder or other medical condition. Sleep disorders, including sleep apnea (that is, absence of breathing during sleep), insomnia, and narcolepsy, may require behavioral, pharmacological, or even surgical intervention to relieve the symptoms.[6, 7] Extra sleep may not eliminate daytime sleepiness that may be due to such disorders.

✎ What's It Mean?

Biological Clock: A collection of cells that regulates an overt biological rhythm, such as the sleep/wake cycle, or some other aspect of biological timing, including reproductive cycles or hibernation.

Source: Copyright © 2003 by BSCS.

Functions Of Sleep

Animal studies have demonstrated that sleep is essential for survival. Consider studies that have been performed with laboratory rats. While these animals will normally live for two to three years, rats deprived of REM sleep survive an average of only five months. Rats deprived of all sleep survive only about three weeks.[1] In humans, extreme sleep deprivation can cause an apparent state of paranoia and hallucinations in otherwise healthy individuals. However, despite identifying several physiological changes that occur in the brain and body during sleep, scientists still do not fully understand the functions of sleep. Many hypotheses have been advanced to explain the role of this necessary and natural behavior.[1] The following examples highlight several of these theories:

Hypothesis: Restoration and recovery of body systems. This theory recognizes the need of an organism to replenish its energy stores and generally repair itself after a period of energy consumption and breakdown (wakefulness). The brain remains active during sleep, and the low metabolic rate characteristic of sleep is thought to be conducive to biosynthetic reactions. There is little, if any, evidence that more repair occurs during sleep than during rest or relaxed wakefulness. In fact, whole-body protein synthesis decreases during sleep, which is consistent with sleep being a period of overnight fasting.

Hypothesis: Energy conservation. This theory states that we sleep to conserve energy and is based on the fact that the metabolic rate is lower during sleep. The theory predicts that total sleep time and NREM sleep time will be proportional to the amount of energy expended during wakefulness. Support for this theory is derived from several lines of evidence. For example, NREM and REM sleep states are found only in endothermic animals (that is, those that expend energy to maintain body temperature). Species with greater total sleep times generally have higher core body temperatures and higher metabolic rates. Consider also that NREM sleep time and total sleep time decrease in humans, with age, as do body and brain metabolism. In addition, infectious diseases tend to make us feel sleepy. This may be because molecules called cytokines, which regulate the function of the immune system, are powerful sleep inducers. It may be that sleep allows the body to conserve energy and other resources, which the immune system may then use to fight the infection.

♣ **It's A Fact!!**

Sleep is an important a part of your health and energy—
it ranks right up there with diet and exercise. Sleep gives you
the energy to play video games and basketball, and to study. Even if
you could study for 9 hours straight without getting tired, you'll remember what you studied more if you sleep after studying. While you sleep, your body stores memories. And not sleeping enough can make you clumsy—that's no good while you're on the court. While you sleep, your brain releases the hormones that control your growth. If you don't sleep enough, you may be tired, cranky, klutzy, and forgetful.

While scientists are a little baffled about why all this recharging can happen only when we sleep, they all agree that we do need to sleep.

Source: "Pillow Pitch," BAM! (Body And Mind), Centers
for Disease Control and Prevention (http://
www.bam.gov), 2005.

Hypothesis: Memory consolidation. The idea here is that sleeping reinforces learning and memory, while at the same time, helping us to forget or to clear stores of unneeded memories. During the course of a day we are inundated with experiences, some of which should be remembered while others need not be. Perhaps sleep aids in rearranging all of the experiences and thoughts from the day so that those that are important are stored and those that are not are discarded. A recent study of songbirds suggests that sleep may play an important role in learning.[8] Young birds listened to the songs of adult birds and began to practice and refine their own songs. The scientists were able to monitor the firing of individual brain cells involved with singing. They found that if sleeping birds listened to a recording of their own song, their neurons would later fire in a pattern nearly identical to that of song production though no sound was produced. The researchers speculate that the birds dream of singing; they relay and rehearse their songs and strengthen the nerve patterns required for song production. Sleep appears to be important for human learning as well. People who get plenty of deep NREM sleep in the first half of the night and REM sleep in the second half improve their ability to perform spatial tasks. This suggests that the full night's sleep plays a role in learning—not just one kind of sleep or the other.

Hypothesis: Protection from predation. Inactivity during sleep may minimize exposure to predators. At the same time, however, sleep decreases sensitivity to external stimuli and may, as a consequence, increase vulnerability to predation.

Hypothesis: Brain development. This proposed function of sleep is related to REM sleep, which occurs for prolonged periods during fetal and infant development. This sleep state may be involved in the formation of brain synapses.

Hypothesis: Discharge of emotions. Perhaps dreaming during REM sleep provides a safe discharge of emotions. As protection to ourselves and to a bed partner, the muscular paralysis that occurs during REM sleep does not allow us to act out what we are dreaming. Additionally, activity in brain regions that control emotions, decision making, and social interactions is reduced during sleep. Perhaps this provides relief from the stresses that occur during wakefulness and helps maintain optimal performance when awake.

Unfortunately, each of these hypotheses suffers from flaws. Most fail because they cannot offer a mechanism for why sleep is more valuable than simply resting while remaining awake. In others, the shortcomings are more subtle.

Evolution Of Sleep

Sleep is ubiquitous among mammals, birds, and reptiles, although sleep patterns, habits, postures, and places of sleep vary greatly. Consider the following:

- **Sleep Patterns:** Mammals generally alternate between NREM and REM sleep states in a cyclic fashion as described earlier, although the length of the sleep cycle

✎ What's It Mean?

Electroencephalogram (EEG): A measurement of the electrical activity associated with brain activity.

Non-Rapid Eye Movement (NREM) Sleep: The early phase of sleep with no rapid eye movement.

Ubiquitous: Seeming to be everywhere.

Source: Copyright © 2003 by BSCS.

and the percentage of time spent in NREM and REM states vary with the animal. Birds also have NREM/REM cycles, although each phase is very short (NREM sleep is about two and one-half minutes; REM sleep is about nine seconds). Additionally, birds do not lose muscle tone during REM sleep, a good thing for animals that sleep while standing or perching. Most scientific studies have failed to demonstrate REM sleep in reptiles. These findings have led some scientists to suggest that REM sleep may be a later evolutionary development related to warm-blooded animals.

- **Sleep Habits:** Some mammals, such as humans, sleep primarily at night, while other mammals, such as rats, sleep primarily during the day. Furthermore, most (but not all) small mammals tend to sleep more than large ones. In some cases, animals have developed ways to sleep and concurrently satisfy critical life functions. These animals engage in unihemispheric sleep, in which one side of the brain sleeps while the other side is awake. This phenomenon is observed most notably in birds (like those that make long, transoceanic flights) and aquatic mammals (like dolphins and porpoises). Unihemispheric sleep allows aquatic mammals to sleep and continue to swim and surface to breathe. It allows animals to keep track of other group members and watch for predators. In fact, there is recent scientific evidence that mallard ducks can increase their use of unihemispheric sleep as the risk of predation increases.[9]

- **Sleep Postures:** A wide variety of postures are seen: from sleeping curled up (dogs, cats, and many other animals), to standing (horses, birds), swimming (aquatic mammals, ducks), hanging upside down (bats), straddling a tree branch (leopard), and lying down (humans).

- **Sleep Places:** Again, there is great variety, especially for mammals: burrows (rabbits), open spaces (lions), under water (hippopotami), nests (gorillas), and the comfort of one's own bed (humans).

Sleep may also occur among lower life forms, such as fish and invertebrates, but it is hard to know because electroencephalogram (EEG) patterns are not comparable to those of vertebrates. Consequently, investigating sleep in species other than mammals and birds has relied on the identification of specific behavioral characteristics of sleep: a quiet state, a typical species-specific sleep posture, an elevated arousal threshold (or reduced responsiveness to external stimuli), rapid waking due to moderately intense stimulation (that is, sleep is rapidly reversible), and a regulated response to sleep deprivation. Recent research demonstrates that even the fruit fly Drosophila melanogaster responds similarly to mammals when exposed to chemical agents that alter sleep patterns.[10, 11]

Comparative studies have explored the evolution of sleep. Although REM sleep is thought to have evolved from NREM sleep, recent studies suggest that NREM and REM sleep may have diverged from a common precursor sleep state.

Sleep Loss And Wakefulness

About 30 to 40 percent of adults indicate some degree of sleep loss within any given year, and about 10 to 15 percent indicate that their sleep loss is chronic or severe.[16] In addition, millions of Americans experience problems sleeping because of undiagnosed sleep disorders or sleep deprivation. Adolescents and shift workers are at very high risk of problem sleepiness

Table 1.1. Representative Total Sleep Requirements For Various Species

Species	Average Total Sleep Time (hours/day)
brown bat	19.9
python	18.0
owl monkey	17.0
human infant	16.0
tiger	15.8
squirrel	14.9
golden hamster	14.3
lion	13.5
gerbil	13.1
rat	12.6
cat	12.1
mouse	12.1
rabbit	11.4
jaguar	10.8
duck	10.8
dog	10.6
bottle-nosed dolphin	10.4
baboon	10.3
chimpanzee	9.7
guinea pig	9.4
human adolescent	9.0
human adult	8.0
pig	7.8
gray seal	6.2
goat	5.3
cow	3.9
sheep	3.8
elephant	3.5
donkey	3.1
horse	2.9
giraffe	1.9

Sources: References 12, 13, 14, and 15.

> **✎ What's It Mean?**
>
> Thermoregulation: Maintenance of internal body temperature regardless of environmental temperature.
>
> Source: Copyright © 2003 by BSCS.

due to sleep deprivation and the desynchronized timing of sleep and wakefulness, respectively.

Sleep and wakefulness are linked in part to the activity of the circadian clock. Recent studies show that individual preferences for morning and evening activity may have a biological basis.[17] In addition, studies show that adolescents experience a delay in the circadian timing system that results in a tendency for them to stay up later and sleep in later.[18] Loss of sleep creates an overwhelming and uncontrollable need to sleep and affects virtually all physiological functions. Sleep loss causes problems with memory and attention, complex thought, motor responses to stimuli, performance in school or on the job, and controlling emotions. Sleep loss may also alter thermoregulation and increase the risk for various physical and mental disorders.

Sleep loss affects personal safety on the road. The National Highway Traffic Safety Administration has estimated that approximately 100,000 motor vehicle crashes each year result from a driver's drowsiness or fatigue while at the wheel.[3] Driving at night or in the early to mid afternoon increases the risk of a crash because those are times that our biological clocks make us sleepy. Drowsy driving impairs a driver's reaction time, vigilance, and ability to make sound judgments. Many adolescents are chronically sleep-deprived and hence at high risk of drowsy-driving crashes. In one large study of fall-asleep crashes, over 50 percent occurred with a driver 25 years old or younger.

References

1. Rechtschaffen, A. 1998. Current perspectives on the function of sleep. *Perspectives in Biological Medicine*, 41: 359–390.

2. Strohl, K.P., Haponik, E.E., Sateia, M.J., Veasey, S., Chervin, R.D., Zee, P., and Papp, K. 2000. The need for a knowledge system in sleep and chronobiology. *Academic Medicine*, 75: 819–21.

3. National Highway Traffic Safety Administration. 1998. Drowsy driving and automobile crashes. Retrieved July 13, 2000, from http://www.sleep foundation.org/activities/ daaafacts.html.

4. Pack, A.I., Pack, A.M., Rodgman, E., Cucchiara, A., Dinges, D.F., and Schwab, C.W. 1995. Characteristics of crashes attributed to the driver having fallen asleep. *Accident Analysis and Prevention*, 27: 769–75.

5. Hastings, M. 1998. The brain, circadian rhythms, and clock genes. *British Medical Journal*, 317: 1704–1707.

6. National Heart, Lung, and Blood Institute. 1995. *Insomnia* (NIH Pub. No. 95-3801). Bethesda, MD: NHLBI.

7. National Heart, Lung, and Blood Institute. 1997a. *Problem sleepiness* (NIH Pub. No. 97-4071). Bethesda, MD: NHLBI.

8. Dave, A.S., and Margoliash, D. 2000. Song replay during sleep and computational rules for sensoring vocal learning. *Science*, 290: 812–816.

9. Rattenborg, N.C., Lima, S.L., and Amlaner, C.J. 1999. Half-awake to the risk of predation. *Nature*, 397: 397–398.

10. Hendricks, J.C., Finn, S.M., Panckeri, K.A., Chavkin, J., Williams, J.A., Sehgal, A., and Pack, A.I. 2000. Rest in Drosophila is a sleep-like state. *Neuron*, 25: 129–138.

11. Shaw, P.J., Cirelli, C., Greenspan, R., and Tononi, G. 2000. Correlates of sleep and waking in *Drosophila melanogaster*. *Science*, 287: 1834–1837.

12. Aserinsky, E. 1999. Eyelid condition at birth: relationship to adult mammalian sleep-waking patterns. In B.N. Mallick and S. Inoue, Eds. *Rapid Eye Movement Slee*p (p. 7). New Delhi: Naroca Publishing.

13. Campbell, S.S., and Tobler, I. 1984. Animal sleep: a review of sleep duration across phylogeny. *Neuroscience and Biobehavioral Review*, 8: 269–300.

14. Kryger, M.H., Roth, Y., and Dement, W.C. 1989. *Principles and Practice of Sleep Medicine*. Philadelphia, PA: W.B. Saunders.

15. Tobler, I. 1989. Napping and polyphasic sleep in mammals. In D.F. Dinges and R.J. Broughton, Eds. *Sleep Alertness: Chronological, Behavioral, and Medical Aspects of Napping* (pp. 9–31). New York: Raven Press.

16. Mellinger, G.D., Balter M.B., and Uhlenhuth, E.H. 1985. Insomnia and its treatment, prevalence and correlates. *Archives of General Psychiatry*, 42: 225–232.

17. Toh, K.L., Jones, C.R., He, Y., Eide, E.J., Hinz, W.A., Virshup, D.M., Ptacek, L.J., and Fu, Y.H. 2001. An h*Per2* phosphorylation site mutation in familial advanced sleep phase syndrome. *Science*, 291: 1040–1043.

18. Carskadon, M.A., Acebo C., Richardson, G.S., Tate, B.A., and Seifer, R. 1997. An approach to studying circadian rhythms of adolescent humans. *Journal of Biological Rhythms*, 12: 278–289.

Chapter 2

The Biology Of Sleep

Research is providing a scientific foundation for understanding sleep's physiology, rhythms, and implications for our health. Although much remains to be learned, this research is clarifying a number of important issues relating to sleep.

Sleep Is A Dynamic Process

Sleep is not a passive event, but rather an active process involving characteristic physiological changes in the organs of the body. Scientists study sleep by measuring the electrical changes in the brain using electroencephalograms (EEGs). Typically, electrodes are placed on the scalp in a symmetrical pattern. The electrodes measure very small voltages that scientists think are caused by synchronized activity in very large numbers of synapses (nerve connections) in the brain's outer layers (cerebral cortex). EEG data are represented by curves that are classified according to their frequencies. The wavy lines of the EEG are called brain waves. An electrooculogram (EOG) uses electrodes on the skin near the eye to measure changes in voltage as the eye rotates in its socket. Scientists also measure the electrical activity associated with active muscles by using electromyograms (EMGs). In this technique, electrodes are placed on the skin overlaying a muscle. In humans, the electrodes are placed under the chin because muscles in this area demonstrate very dramatic changes during the various stages of sleep.

✎ What's It Mean?

Amplitude: Magnitude, greatness of size.

Electroencephalograms (EEGs): A measurement of the electrical activity associated with brain activity.

Electromyograms (EMGs): A measurement of the electrical activity associated with muscle movements.

Electrooculogram (EOG): A measurement of the electrical activity associated with eye movements.

Frequency: The number of times a periodic process occurs per unit of time.

Non-Rapid Eye Movement (NREM) Sleep: The early phase of sleep with no rapid eye movement.

Rapid Eye Movement (REM) Sleep: Deep sleep with rapid eye movements in which dreaming takes place.

Source: Copyright © 2003 by BSCS.

In practice, EEGs, EOGs, and EMGs are recorded simultaneously on continuously moving chart paper or digitized by a computer and displayed on a high-resolution monitor. This allows the relationships among the three measurements to be seen immediately. The patterns of activity in these three systems provide the basis for classifying the different types of sleep.

Studying these events has led to the identification of two basic stages, or states, of sleep: non-rapid eye movement (NREM) and rapid eye movement (REM).[1,2]

Sleep is a highly organized sequence of events that follows a regular, cyclic program each night. Thus, the EEG, EMG, and EOG patterns change in predictable ways several times during a single sleep period. NREM sleep is divided into four stages according to the amplitude and frequency of brain wave activity. In general, the EEG pattern of NREM sleep is slower, often more regular, and usually of higher voltage than that of wakefulness. As sleep gets deeper, the brain waves get slower and have greater amplitude. NREM Stage 1 is very light sleep; NREM Stage 2 has special brain waves called sleep spindles and K complexes; NREM Stages 3 and 4 show increasingly more high voltage slow waves. In NREM Stage 4, it is extremely hard to be awakened by external stimuli. The muscle activity of NREM sleep is low, but the muscles retain their ability to function. Eye movements normally do not occur during NREM sleep, except for very slow eye movements, usually at the beginning. The body's general physiology during these stages is fairly similar to the wake state. In this chapter, NREM sleep is represented in general and not its individual substages.

The EEG recorded during REM sleep shows very fast and desynchronized activity that is more random than that recorded during NREM sleep. It actually looks similar to the EEG (low voltage with a faster mix of frequencies) from when we are awake. REM sleep is characterized by bursts of rapid eye movements. The eyes are not constantly moving, but they dart back and forth or up and down. They also stop for a while and then jerk back and

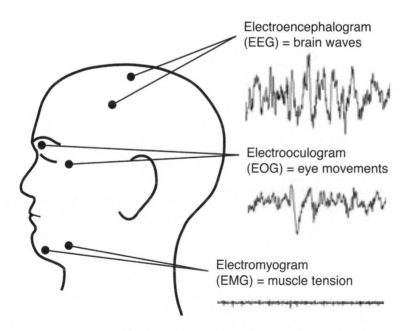

Electroencephalogram
(EEG) = brain waves

Electrooculogram
(EOG) = eye movements

Electromyogram
(EMG) = muscle tension

Figure 2.1. Placement of electrodes to determine EEG, EOG, and EMG.

forth again. Always, and just like waking eye movements, both eyes move together in the same direction. Some scientists believe that the eye movements of REM sleep relate to the visual images of dreams, but why they exist and what function they serve, if any, remain unknown. Additionally, while muscle tone is normal in NREM sleep, we are almost completely paralyzed in REM sleep. Although the muscles that move our bodies go limp, other important muscles continue to function in REM sleep. These include the heart, diaphragm, eye muscles, and smooth muscles such as those of the intestines and blood vessels. The paralysis of muscles in the arms and legs and under the chin show electrical silence in REM sleep. On an EMG, the recording produces a flat line. Small twitches can break through this paralysis and look like tiny blips on the flat line.

Sleep is a cyclical process. During sleep, people experience repeated cycles of NREM and REM sleep, beginning with an NREM phase. This cycle lasts approximately 90 to 110 minutes and is repeated four to six times per night. As the night progresses, however, the amount of deep NREM sleep decreases and the amount of REM sleep increases. The term ultradian rhythm

✎ What's It Mean?

Anesthesia: Complete or partial loss of sensation, usually caused by artificially produced unconsciousness.

Follicle Stimulating Hormone: A hormone produced in the pituitary gland that stimulates the growth of follicles in the ovary and induces spermatogenesis in the testes.

Hypnogram: A graphical summary of the electrical activities occurring during a night's sleep.

Luteinizing Hormone: A glycoprotein secreted by the pituitary gland. It stimulates the gonads to secrete sex steroids.

Ultradian Rhythm: A periodicity of less than 24 hours.

Source: Copyright © 2003 by BSCS.

(that is, rhythm occurring within a period of less than 24 hours) is used to describe this cycling through sleep stages.

The chart in Figure 2.2 is called a hypnogram. Hypnograms were developed to summarize the voluminous chart recordings of electrical activities (EEG, EOG, and EMG) collected during a night's sleep. Hypnograms provide a simple way to display information originally collected on many feet of chart paper or stored as a large file on a computer.

We can make several observations about the hypnogram in Figure 2.2. First, the periods of NREM and REM sleep alternate during the night. Second, the deepest stages of NREM sleep occur in the first part of the night. Third, the episodes of REM sleep are longer as the night progresses. This hypnogram also indicates two periods during the night when the individual awakened (at about six and seven hours into the night).

It is useful to distinguish between sleep and the state induced during general anesthesia or seen in people who are in a coma. While these latter individuals are often said to be "asleep," their conditions are not readily reversible (that is, they cannot be awakened by a strong stimulus), and they do not exhibit the same brain wave patterns characteristic of true sleep.

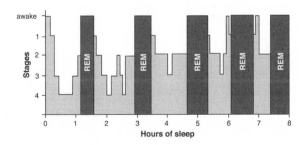

Figure 2.2. A typical hypnogram from a young, healthy adult. Light-gray areas represent non-rapid eye movement (NREM) sleep.

Physiological Changes During Sleep

Table 2.1 summarizes some basic physiological changes that occur in NREM and REM sleep.

The functions of many organ systems are also linked to the sleep cycle, as follows:

- **Endocrine System:** Most hormone secretion is controlled by the circadian clock or in response to physical events. Sleep is one of the events that modify the timing of secretion for certain hormones. Many hormones are secreted into the blood during sleep. For example, scientists believe that the release of growth hormone is related in part to repair processes that occur during sleep. Follicle stimulating hormone and luteinizing hormone, which are involved in maturational and reproductive processes, are among the hormones released during sleep. In fact, the sleep-dependent release of luteinizing hormone is thought to be the event that initiates puberty. Other hormones, such as thyroid-stimulating hormone, are released prior to sleep.

- **Renal System:** Kidney filtration, plasma flow, and the excretion of sodium, chloride, potassium, and calcium all are reduced during both NREM and REM sleep. These changes cause urine to be more concentrated during sleep.

- **Alimentary Activity:** In a person with normal digestive function, gastric acid secretion is reduced during sleep. In those with an active ulcer, gastric acid secretion is actually increased. In addition, swallowing occurs less frequently.

Sleep And The Brain

Sleep is actively generated in specific brain regions. These sites have been identified through studies involving electrical stimulation, damage to specific brain regions, or other techniques that identify sleep-inducing sites. The basal forebrain, including the hypothalamus, is an important region for controlling NREM sleep and may be the region keeping track of how long we have been awake and how large our sleep debt is. The brainstem region known as the pons is critical for initiating REM sleep. As depicted in Figure

2.3, during REM sleep, the pons sends signals to the visual nuclei of the thalamus and to the cerebral cortex (this region is responsible for most of our thought processes). The pons also sends signals to the spinal cord, causing the temporary paralysis that is characteristic of REM sleep. Other brain sites are also important in the sleep process. For example, the thalamus generates many of the brain rhythms in NREM sleep that we see as EEG patterns.

Table 2.1. Comparison Of Physiological Changes During NREM And REM Sleep

Physiological Process	During NREM	During REM
brain activity	decreases from wakefulness	increases in motor and sensory areas, while other areas are similar to NREM
heart rate	slows from wakefulness	increases and varies compared with NREM
blood pressure	decreases from wakefulness	increases (up to 30 percent) and varies from NREM
blood flow to brain	does not change from wakefulness in most regions	increases by 50 to 200 percent from NREM, depending on brain region
respiration	decreases from wakefulness	increases and varies from NREM, but may show brief stoppages (apnea); coughing suppressed
airway resistance	increases from wakefulness	increases and varies from wakefulness
body temperature	is regulated at lower set point than wakefulness; shivering initiated at lower temperature than during wakefulness	is not regulated; no shivering or sweating; temperature drifts toward that of the local environment
sexual arousal	occurs infrequently	increases from NREM (in both males and females)

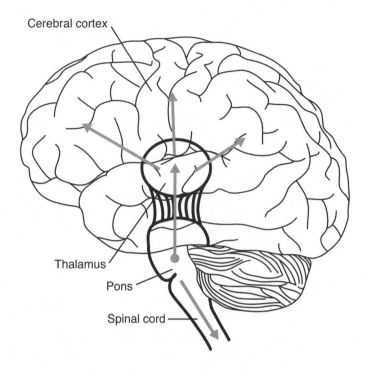

Figure 2.3. Pathways of brain activity during REM sleep.

References

1. Kohyama, J. 1998. Sleep as a window on the developing brain. *Current Problems in Pediatrics*, 27: 73–92.

2. University of California and Sleep Research Society. 1997. Basics of sleep behavior. Retrieved July 17, 2001, from http://www.sleephomepages.org/sleepsyllabus.

✎ What's It Mean?

Cerebral Cortex: The brain's outer layer of gray tissue that is responsible for higher nervous function.

Hypothalamus: The part of the brain that lies below the thalamus and regulates body temperature and metabolic processes.

Pons: The brainstem region critical for initiating REM sleep.

Thalamus: The area of the brain that relays sensory information to the cerebral cortex.

Source: Copyright © 2003 by BSCS.

Chapter 3
Sleep Patterns And Circadian Rhythms

Sleep Patterns

Sleep patterns change during an individual's life. In fact, age affects sleep more than any other natural factor. Newborns sleep an average of 16 to 18 hours per day. By the time a child is three to five years old, total sleep time averages 10 to 12 hours, and then it further decreases to 7 to 8 hours per night by adulthood. One of the most prominent age-related changes in sleep is a reduction in the time spent in the deepest stages of NREM (Stages 3 and 4) from childhood through adulthood. In fact, this change is prominent during adolescence, when about 40 percent of this activity is lost and replaced by Stage 2 NREM sleep. In addition to these changes, the percentage of time spent in REM sleep also changes during development. Newborns may spend about 50 percent of their total sleep time in REM sleep. In fact, unlike older children and adults, infants fall asleep directly into REM sleep. Infant sleep cycles generally last only 50 to 60 minutes. By two years of age, REM sleep accounts for 20 to 25 percent of total sleep time, which remains relatively constant throughout the remainder of life.[1] Young children have a high arousal threshold, which means they can sleep through loud noises, especially in the early part of the night. For example, one study showed that 10-year-olds were undisturbed by a noise as loud as the sound of a jet airplane taking off nearby.

♣ It's A Fact!!

Sleep is divided into five stages. The sleep stages come in cycles. All night, we go through a series of cycles that last about 90 minutes.

Stages 1 And 2

Light sleep. In fact, stage 1 sleep is very close to being very relaxed when you're awake. It's easier to wake up or be woken up. If you wake up in these phases, you might not even realize you were asleep.

Stages 3 And 4

Deep sleep. Your breathing and heart rate slow down. The deeper the sleep, the better it is for you. It's hard to wake up from stages 3 and 4. You might feel groggy or not realize what's going on at first.

REM

REM is short for "rapid eye movement." This stage is when you dream. If you remember a dream, it's probably because you were in REM sleep when you woke up. You can tell when someone's in the stage because their eyes move around, even though they're closed, like they're looking at everything in their dream. The brain sends out signals to the rest of your muscles to keep them from acting out your dreams. Sometimes, the signals don't work. That's when some people might talk or walk in their sleep. Scientists don't know yet why that happens.

Source: "Pillow Pitch: Under the Microscope," BAM! (Body and Mind), Centers for Disease Control and Prevention, 2005.

Although most humans maintain REM sleep throughout life, brain disorders like Alzheimer disease and Parkinson disease are characterized by decreasing amounts of REM sleep as the diseases progress. Also, elderly individuals exhibit more variation in the duration and quality of sleep than do younger adults. Elderly people may also exhibit increased sleep fragmentation (arousals from sleep that occur as either short or more extended awakenings). Figure 3.1 depicts these developmental changes in sleep patterns.

Several issues are important to consider. First, individual sleep needs vary. For instance, eight hours of sleep per night appears to be optimal for most adults, although some may need more or less. Teenagers, on average, require about nine or more hours of sleep per night to be as alert as possible when awake. If sleep needs are not met, a bioprogressive sleep debt occurs and eventually the body requires that the debt be paid. It does not appear that we are able to adapt to getting less sleep than our bodies require. Not getting enough sleep, while still allowing us to function in a seemingly normal manner, does impair motor and cognitive functions. Caffeine and other stimulants cannot substitute for sleep, but they do help counteract some of the effects of sleep deprivation.

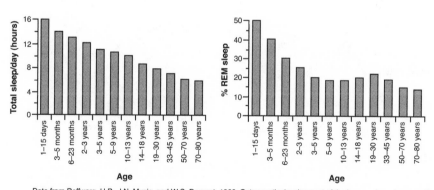

Data from Roffwarg, H.P., J.N. Muzic, and W.C. Dement. 1966. Ontogenetic development of the human sleep-dream cycle. *Science*, 152: 604–619.

Figure 3.1. Average sleep need (left graph) and percentage of REM sleep (right graph) at different ages.

Biological Clock

An internal biological clock regulates the timing for sleep in humans. The activity of this clock makes us sleepy at night and awake during the day. Our clock cycles with an approximately 24-hour period and is called a circadian clock (from the Latin roots *circa* = about and *diem* = day). In humans, this clock is located in the suprachiasmatic nucleus (SCN) of the hypothalamus in the brain.[2] The SCN is actually a very small structure consisting of a pair of pinhead-size regions, each containing only about 10,000 neurons out of the brain's estimated 100 billion neurons.

Biological clocks are genetically programmed physiological systems that allow organisms to live in harmony with natural rhythms, such as day/night cycles and the changing of seasons. The most important function of a

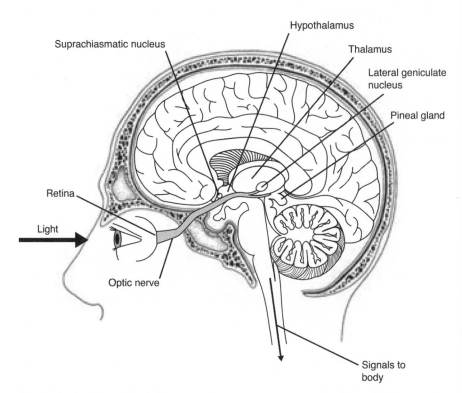

Figure 3.2. The biological clock is located within the suprachiasmatic nucleus in the brain.

biological clock is to regulate overt biological rhythms like the sleep/wake cycle. The biological clock is also involved in controlling seasonal reproductive cycles in some animals through its ability to track information about the changing lengths of daylight and darkness during a year. Biological rhythms are of two general types. Exogenous rhythms are directly produced by an external influence, such as an environmental cue. They are not generated internally by the organism itself, and if the environmental cues are removed, the rhythm ceases. Endogenous rhythms, by contrast, are driven by an internal, self-sustaining biological clock rather than by anything external to the organism. Biological rhythms, such as oscillations in core body temperature, are endogenous. They are maintained even if environmental cues are removed.

Because the circadian clock in most humans has a natural day length of just over 24 hours, the clock must be entrained, or reset, to match the day length of the environmental photoperiod (that is, the light/dark, or day/night, cycle). The cue that synchronizes the internal biological clock to the environmental cycle is light. Photoreceptors in the retina transmit light-dependent signals to the SCN. Interestingly, our usual visual system receptors, the rods and cones, are apparently not required for this photoreception.[3] Special types of retinal ganglion cells are photoreceptive, project directly to the SCN, and appear to have all the properties required to provide the light signals for synchronizing the biological clock.[4] At the SCN, the signal interacts with several genes that serve as "pacemakers."

✎ What's It Mean?

Circadian: Exhibiting a periodicity of 24 hours.

Endogenous Rhythms: Rhythms driven by an internal, self-sustaining biological clock rather than by signals that are external to the organism (for example, light).

Exogenous Rhythms: A rhythm that is directly regulated by an external influence, such as an environmental cue. They are not generated internally by the organism itself.

Oscillation: The state or act of swinging back and forth with a regular, uninterrupted pattern.

Suprachiasmatic Nucleus (SCN): The part of the brain (in the hypothalamus) that contains the biological clock.

Source: Copyright © 2003 by BSCS.

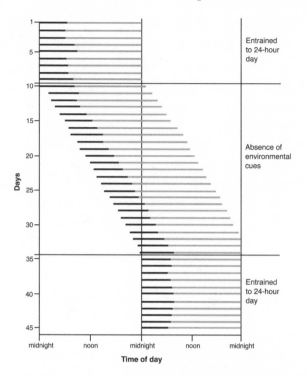

Figure 3.3. Entrainment of the biological clock. Black bars, asleep; gray bars, awake.

Endogenous sleep rhythms can be depicted graphically. Figure 3.3 shows a day-by-day representation of one individual's sleep/wake cycle. The black lines indicate periods of sleep, and the gray lines indicate periods of wakefulness. The upper portion of the figure (days 1 through 9) represents this individual's normal sleep/wake cycle. Under these conditions, the individual is exposed to regularly timed exposure to alternating daylight and darkness, which has entrained this person's sleep/wake cycling to a period of 24 hours.

Contrast this upper portion of the figure with the middle portion (days 10 through 34). In the middle portion, this individual has been isolated from normal environmental cues like daylight, darkness, temperature variation, and noise variation. There are two important points to be derived from this portion of the figure. First, this individual's sleep/wake cycle continues to oscillate in the absence of external cues, stressing that this rhythm is endogenous, or built in. Second, in the absence of external cues to entrain circadian rhythms, this individual's clock cycles with its own natural, built-in rhythm that is just over 24 hours long. Consequently, without environmental cues, the individual goes to bed about one hour later each night. After 24 days, the individual is once again going to bed at midnight. The lower portion of Figure 3.3 depicts the change in the sleep/wake cycle after the individual is once again entrained to a 24-hour day containing the proper environmental cues.

Another interesting rhythm that is controlled by the biological clock is the cycle of body temperature, which is lowest in the biological night and rises in the biological daytime. This fluctuation persists even in the absence of sleep. Activity during the day and sleep during the night reinforce this cycle of changes in body temperature.

The release of melatonin, a hormone produced by the pineal gland, is controlled by the circadian clock in the SCN. Its levels rise during the night and decline at dawn in both nocturnal and diurnal species. Melatonin has been called the hormone of darkness because of this pattern. The SCN controls the timing of melatonin release; melatonin then feeds back on the SCN to regulate its activity. In mammals, for example, most of the brain receptors for melatonin are located in the SCN. Research has demonstrated that administering melatonin can produce shifts in circadian rhythms in a number of species including rats, sheep, lizards, birds, and humans. These effects are

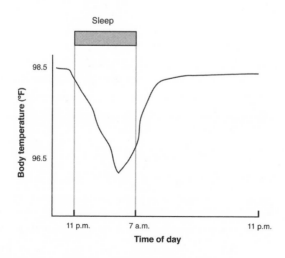

Figure 3.4. Body temperature in relation to the sleep cycle.

most clearly evident when melatonin is given in the absence of light
input. Thus, for example, giving
melatonin to blind people can help
set their biological clocks. Melatonin is available as an over-the-
counter nutritional supplement.
Although claims are made that the
supplement promotes sleep, the evidence for this is inconclusive. Potential side effects of long-term
administration of melatonin remain
unknown, and its unsupervised use
by the general public is discouraged.

In addition to synchronizing
these daily rhythms, biological
clocks can affect rhythms that are

✎ What's It Mean?

Cytoplasm: Protoplasm outside a
cell nucleus.

Diurnal: Active or occurring during the daytime; repeating once
each 24 hours.

Melatonin: A hormone secreted by
the pineal gland that is derived
from the amino acid tryptophan,
which helps synchronize biological clock neurons in the
suprachiasmatic nucleus.

Nocturnal: Relating to or taking
place at night.

Source: Copyright © 2003 by BSCS.

longer than 24 hours, especially seasonal rhythms. Some vertebrates have
reproductive systems that are sensitive to day length. These animals can sense
changes in day length by the amount of melatonin secreted. The short days
and long nights of winter turn off the reproductive systems of hamsters,
while in sheep the opposite occurs. The high levels of melatonin that inhibit
reproduction in hamsters stimulate the reproductive systems of sheep, so
they breed in winter and give birth in the spring.

Biological clocks exist in a wide range of organisms, from *Cyanobacteria*
(blue-green algae) to humans. Clocks enable organisms to adapt to their
surroundings. Although scientists currently believe that clocks arose through
independent evolution and may use different clock proteins, they all share
several regulatory characteristics. In particular, they are maintained by a biochemical process known as a negative feedback loop.

Much of what is known about clock regulation has come from studying
the fruit fly *Drosophila melanogaster*, from which biological clock genes were
first cloned. Two genes called *period (per)* and *timeless (tim)* were found to
cycle with a 24-hour, or circadian, rhythm.[5, 6] The genes are active early in

the night and produce mRNA that is then translated into the proteins PER and TIM. These proteins begin to accumulate in the cytoplasm. After the proteins have reached high enough levels, PER protein binds to TIM protein, forming a complex that enters the cell's nucleus. In the nucleus, the PER-TIM complexes bind to the *per* and *tim* genes to suppress further transcription. This creates what is called a negative feedback loop. After a while, the PER and TIM proteins degrade, and transcription from the *per* and *tim* genes begins again.

This description of *Drosophila's* clock is a simplified one. Other genes have been identified that produce proteins involved with regulating the circadian clock. For example, the proteins CLOCK, CYCLE, and VRILLE are transcription factors that regulate expression of the *per* and *tim* genes. Other proteins, like the enzymes DOUBLE-TIME and SHAGGY, can alter the periodicity of the clock through chemical modification (phosphorylation) of PER and TIM. Mutations have been identified in clock genes that speed up, slow down, or eliminate the periodicity of the circadian clock in flies. Interestingly, similar genes and proteins have been identified in mammals, and studies indicate that the mammalian clock is regulated in much the same way as that of the fly.[5, 7, 8, 9] Developmental changes in the circadian clock occur from infancy to childhood to adolescence, and further changes occur as adults age. Very little is known about specific genes and mediators responsible for the normal development of the circadian clock.

One negative consequence of our circadian cycle afflicts travelers who rapidly cross multiple time zones. Jet lag produces a number of unwanted effects including excessive sleepiness, poor sleep, loss of concentration, poor motor control, slowed reflexes, nausea, and irritability. Jet lag results from the inability of our circadian clock to make an immediate adjustment to the changes in light cues that an individual experiences when rapidly crossing time zones. After such travel, the body is in conflict. The biological clock carries the rhythm entrained by the original time zone, even though the clock is out of step with the cues in the new time zone. This conflict between external and internal clocks and signals is called desynchronization, and it affects more than just the sleep/wake cycle. All the rhythms are out of sync, and they take a number of days to re-entrain to the new time zone. Eastward

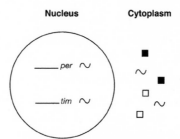

Nucleus   **Cytoplasm**

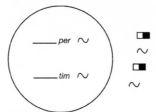

a. Early in the night, the *per* and *tim* genes are active producing mRNA
(~) that moves to the cytoplasm to be translated into PER (■) and
TIM (□) proteins.

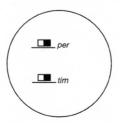

b. The PER and TIM proteins bind to each other to form a complex (□■)
that enters the nucleus.

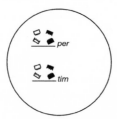

c. The PER-TIM complexes bind to the *per* and *tim* genes,
stopping their transcription.

d. Eventually, the PER-TIM complexes break down and the *per*
and *tim* genes become active again.

Figure 3.5. In the fruit fly, the biological clock is largely controlled by two genes called
per *and* tim, *whose expression cycles with an approximately 24-hour period. This
cycling of gene expression is controlled by a process called a negative feedback loop.*

travel generally causes more severe jet lag than westward travel, because traveling east requires that we shorten our day and adjust to time cues occurring earlier than our clock is used to. In general, the human circadian clock appears better able to adjust to a longer day than a shorter day. For example, it is easier for most people to adjust to the end of daylight savings time in the fall when we have one 25-hour day than to the start of daylight savings time in the spring, when we have a 23-hour day. Similarly, traveling from the West Coast of the United States to the East Coast produces a loss of three hours—a 21-hour day. Thus, travelers may find it difficult to sleep because of the three-hour difference between external cues and their internal clock. Likewise, travelers may find it difficult to awaken in the morning. We may try to go to sleep and wake up at our usual local times of, say, 11 P.M. and 7 A.M., but to our brain's biological clock, the times are 8 P.M. and 4 A.M. Other circadian rhythm problems include:

- **Monday Morning Blues:** By staying up and sleeping in an hour or more later than usual on the weekends, we provide our biological clock different cues that push it toward a later nighttime phase. By keeping a late sleep schedule both weekend nights, our internal clock becomes two hours or more behind our usual weekday schedule. When the alarm rings at 6:30 A.M. on Monday, our body's internal clock is now set for 4:30 A.M. or earlier.

- **Seasonal Affective Disorder (SAD):** A change of seasons in autumn brings on both a loss of daylight savings time (fall back one hour) and a shortening of the daytime. As winter progresses, the day length becomes even shorter. During this season of short days and long nights, some individuals develop symptoms similar to jet lag but more severe. These symptoms include decreased appetite, loss of concentration and focus, lack of energy, feelings of depression and despair, and excessive sleepiness. Too little bright light reaching the biological clock in the SCN appears to bring on this recognized form of depression in susceptible individuals. Consequently, treatment often involves using light therapy.

- **Shift Work:** Unlike some animals, humans are active during daylight hours. This pattern is called diurnal activity. Animals that are awake and active at night (for example, hamsters) have what is known as nocturnal activity. For humans and other diurnally active animals, light signals the time to awake, and sleep occurs during the dark. Modern society, however, requires that services and businesses be available 24 hours a day, so some individuals must work the night shift. These individuals no longer have synchrony between their internal clocks and external daylight and darkness signals, and they may experience mental and physical difficulties similar to jet lag and SAD.

Homeostasis And Sleep

The relationship of circadian rhythms to sleep is relatively well understood. Continuing studies in genetics and molecular biology promise further advances in our knowledge of how the circadian clock works and how a succession of behavioral states adapt to changes in light/dark cycles. In addition to the circadian component, there is a fundamental regulatory process involved in programming sleep. Consider that the longer an individual remains awake, the stronger the desire and need to sleep become. This pressure to sleep defines the homeostatic component of sleep. The precise mechanism underlying the pressure that causes us to feel a need to sleep remains a mystery. What science does know is that the action of nerve-signaling molecules called neurotransmitters and of nerve cells (neurons) located in the brainstem and at the base of the brain determines whether we are asleep or awake. Additionally, there is recent evidence that the molecule adenosine (composed of the base adenine linked to the five-

---

✎ What's It Mean?

Homeostasis: The ability or tendency of an organism or cell to maintain internal equilibrium by adjusting its internal processes.

Homeostatic Regulation Of Sleep: Refers to the neurobiological signals mediating the pressure or urge to sleep.

Neurotransmitters: A chemical produced by neurons that carries messages to other neurons.

Source: Copyright © 2003 by BSCS.

carbon sugar ribose) is an important sleepiness factor: it appears to "keep track" of lost sleep and may induce sleep. Interestingly, caffeine binds to and blocks the same cell receptors that recognize adenosine.[2, 10] This suggests that caffeine disrupts sleep by binding to adenosine receptors and preventing adenosine from delivering its fatigue signal. The homeostatic regulation of sleep helps reinforce the circadian cycle. We usually sleep once daily because the homeostatic pressure to sleep is hard to resist after about 16 hours, and then while we sleep, our closed eyes block the light signals to the biological clock.

♣ It's A Fact!!

While you sleep, your brain stores what you learned during the day before. This means that the next day, you can remember what you learned, pay attention and concentrate, and solve problems and think of new ideas.

Your brain also releases hormones that control how you grow. While you sleep, your muscles, bones, and skin heal and grow, and your immune system gears up in case you need to fight off an illness.

Source: "Pillow Pitch: Under the Microscope," BAM! (Body and Mind), Centers for Disease Control and Prevention, 2005.

References

1. Kohyama, J. 1998. Sleep as a window on the developing brain. *Current Problems in Pediatrics*, 27: 73–92.

2. Moore, R.Y. 1997. Circadian rhythms: Basic neurobiology and clinical applications. *Annual Review of Medicine*, 48: 253–266.

3. Freedman, M.S., Lucas, R.J., Soni, B., von Schantz, M., Munoz, M., David-Gray, Z., and Foster, R. 1999. Regulation of mammalian circadian behavior by non-rod, noncone, ocular photoreceptors. *Science*, 284: 502–504.

4. Berson, D.M., Dunn, F.A., and Takao, M. 2002. Phototransduction by retinal ganglion cells that set the circadian clock. *Science*, 295: 1070–73.

5. Dunlap, J.C. 1999. Molecular bases for circadian clocks. *Cell*, 96: 271–290.

6. Hastings, M. 1998. The brain, circadian rhythms, and clock genes. *British Medical Journal*, 317: 1704–1707.

7. Green, C. 1998. How cells tell time. *Trends in Cell Biology*, 8: 224–230.

8. Hall, J.C. 1997. Circadian pacemakers blowing hot and cold—but they're clocks, not thermometers. *Cell*, 90: 9–12.

9. Reppert, S.M. 1998. A clockwork explosion! *Neuron*, 21: 1–4.

10. Phillis, J.W., and Wu, P.H. 1982. The effect of various centrally active drugs on adenosine uptake by the central nervous system. *Comparative Biochemistry & Physiology, Part C, Pharmacology, Toxicology, and Endocrinology*, 72: 179–187.

Chapter 4

Napping

More than 85% of mammalian species are polyphasic sleepers, meaning that they sleep for short periods throughout the day. Humans are part of the minority of monophasic sleepers, meaning that our days are divided into two distinct periods, one for sleep and one for wakefulness. It is not clear that this is the natural sleep pattern of humans. Young children and elderly persons nap, for example, and napping is a very important aspect of many cultures.

As a nation, the United States appears to be becoming more and more sleep deprived. And it may be our busy lifestyle that keeps us from napping. While naps do not necessarily make up for inadequate or poor quality nighttime sleep, a short nap of 20–30 minutes can help to improve mood, alertness, and performance. Nappers are in good company: Winston Churchill, John F. Kennedy, Ronald Reagan, Napoleon, Albert Einstein, Thomas Edison, and George W. Bush are known to have valued an afternoon nap.

Types Of Naps

Naps can be typed in three different ways:

- Planned napping (also called preparatory napping) involves taking a nap before you actually get sleepy. You may use this technique when you know that you will be up later than your normal bed time or as a mechanism to ward off getting tired earlier.

- Emergency napping occurs when you are suddenly very tired and cannot continue with the activity you were originally engaged in. This type of nap can be used to combat drowsy driving or fatigue while using heavy and dangerous machinery.

- Habitual napping is practiced when a person takes a nap at the same time each day. Young children may fall asleep at about the same time each afternoon or an adult might take a short nap after lunch each day.

Benefits Of Napping

- Naps can restore alertness, enhance performance, and reduce mistakes and accidents. A study at NASA on sleepy military pilots and astronauts found that a 40-minute nap improved performance by 34% and alertness 100%.

✔ **Quick Tip**
Tips For Good Napping

The Right Length: A short nap is usually recommended (20–30 minutes) for short-term alertness. This type of nap provides significant benefit for improved alertness and performance without leaving you feeling groggy or interfering with nighttime sleep.

The Right Environment: Your surroundings can greatly impact your ability to fall asleep. Make sure that you have a restful place to lie down and that the temperature in the room is comfortable. Try to limit the amount of noise heard and the extent of the light filtering in. While some studies have shown that just spending time in bed can be beneficial, it is better to try to catch some zzz's.

The Right Time: If you take a nap too late in the day, it might affect your nighttime sleep patterns and make it difficult to fall asleep at your regular bedtime. If you try to take it too early in the day, your body may not be ready for more sleep.

- Naps can increase alertness in the period directly following the nap and may extend alertness a few hours later in the day.

- Scheduled napping has also been prescribed for those who are affected by narcolepsy.

- Napping has psychological benefits. A nap can be a pleasant luxury, a mini-vacation. It can provide an easy way to get some relaxation and rejuvenation.

Negative Effects Of Napping

- Sleep inertia is defined as the feeling of grogginess and disorientation that can come with awakening from a deep sleep. While this state usually only lasts for a few minutes to a half-hour, it can be detrimental to those who must perform immediately after waking from a napping period. Post-nap impairment and disorientation is more severe, and can last longer, in people who are sleep deprived or nap for longer periods.

- Napping can also have a negative effect on other sleeping periods. A long nap or a nap taken too late in the day may adversely affect the length and quality of nighttime sleep. If you have trouble sleeping at night, a nap will only amplify problems.

- One study has indicated that napping is associated with increased risk of heart failure in people already at risk.

Obstacles To Overcome

While research has shown that napping is a beneficial way to relieve tiredness, it still has stigmas associated with it.

- Napping indicates laziness, a lack of ambition, and low standards.

- Napping is only for children, the sick, and the elderly.

Though the above statements are false, many segments of the public may still need to be educated on the benefits of napping.

Chapter 5

Dreaming

Dreams

An intriguing occurrence during sleep is dreaming. Although reports of dreaming are most frequent and vivid when an individual is aroused from REM sleep, dreams do occur at sleep onset and during NREM sleep as well.[1] During an average night's sleep, about two hours are spent dreaming, mostly during REM sleep. Although some dreams are memorable because of their extraordinary or bizarre nature, other dreams reflect realistic experiences. Despite this realism, REM dreams are usually novel experiences, like a work of fiction, instead of a replay of actual events. Pre-sleep stimuli do not seem to affect dream content. In fact, the source of the content of any given dream is unknown. REM sleep and dreams are associated with each other, but they are not synonymous. While REM sleep is turned on and off by the pons, two areas in the cerebral hemispheres (areas far from the pons that control higher mental functions) regulate dreaming.

REM sleep and dreaming can be dissociated from one another, as seen after the administration of certain drugs or in cases of brain damage either to the pons (loss of REM sleep but not of dreaming) or to the frontal areas

About This Chapter: This chapter begins with text excerpted from "Sleep, Sleep Disorders, and Biological Rhythms," Copyright © 2003 by BSCS. All rights reserved. Reprinted with permission. Additional text is from "Common Questions about Dreams," © 2003 International Association for the Study of Dreams (www.asdreams.org). Reprinted with permission.

(no dreaming but REM sleep cycle unaffected). Consequently, REM sleep appears to be just one of the triggers for dreaming. Using scanning techniques that assess brain activity, scientists have determined which areas of the brain are active during REM sleep dreaming.[2, 3] These areas are illustrated in Figure 5.1. Brain regions that are inactive during dreaming include those that regulate intelligence, conscious thought, and higher-order reasoning. Higher-order reasoning is that part of brain function responsible for processing experiences into memory and regulating vision while we are awake. The significance of dreaming to one's health and the meaning of dreams remain mysteries.

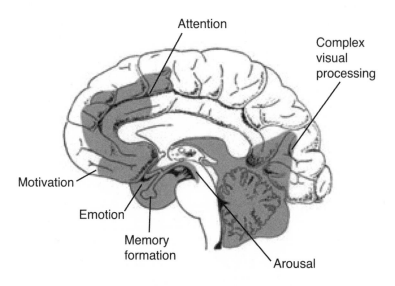

Figure 5.1. Areas of the brain active during REM sleep dreaming.

✎ What's It Mean?

Non-Rapid Eye Movement (NREM) Sleep: The early phase of sleep with no rapid eye movement.

Rapid Eye Movement (REM): Deep sleep with rapid eye movements in which dreaming takes place.

Source: Copyright © 2003 by BSCS.

References

1. National Heart, Lung, and Blood Institute. 1998. *Insomnia: Assessment and management in primary care* (NIH Pub. No. 98-4088). Bethesda, MD: NHLBI.

2. Braun, A.R., Balkin, T.J., and Wesensten, N.L. 1998. Dissociated pattern of activity in visual cortices and their projections during human rapid eye movement sleep. *Science*, 279: 91–95.

3. Hong, C.H., Gillian, J.C., Dow, B.M., et al. 1995. Localized and lateralized cerebral glucose metabolism associated with eye movements during REM sleep and wakefulness: a positron emission tomography (PET) study. *Sleep*, 18: 570–580.

Common Questions About Dreams

Does everyone dream?

Yes. Laboratory studies have shown that we experience our most vivid dreams during a type of sleep called rapid eye movement (REM) sleep. During REM sleep the brain is very active, the eyes move back and forth rapidly under the lids, and the large muscles of the body are relaxed. REM sleep occurs every 90–100 minutes, three to four times a night, and lasts longer as the night progresses. The final REM period may last as long as 45 minutes. Less vivid dreams occur at other times during the night.

Why do people have trouble remembering their dreams?

Some people have no difficulty in remembering several dreams nightly, whereas others recall dreams only occasionally or not at all. Nearly everything that happens during sleep—including dreams, the thoughts which occur throughout the night and memories of brief awakenings—is forgotten by morning. There is something about the phenomenon of sleep itself which makes it difficult to remember what has occurred and most dreams are forgotten unless they are written down. Sometimes a dream is suddenly remembered later in the day or on another day, suggesting that the memory is not totally lost but for some reason is very hard to retrieve. Sleep and dreams also are affected by a great variety of drugs and medications, including alcohol. Further, stopping certain medications suddenly may cause nightmares. It is advisable to discuss with your physician the effect of any drugs or medications you are taking.

Are dreams in color?

Most dreams are in color, although people may not be aware of it, either because they have difficulty remembering their dreams or because color is such a natural part of visual experience. People who are very aware of color while awake probably notice color more often in their dreams.

Do dreams have meaning?

Although scientists continue to debate this issue, most people who work with their dreams, either by themselves or with others, find that their dreams are very meaningful for them. Dreams are useful in learning more about the dreamer's feelings, thoughts, behavior, motives, and values. Many find that dreams can help them solve problems. Further, artists, writers, and scientists often get creative ideas from dreams.

> ✔ **Quick Tip**
>
> *How can I improve my dream memory?*
>
> Before you fall asleep, remind yourself that you want to remember your dreams. Keep a paper and pen or tape-recorder by your bedside. As you awaken, try to move as little as possible and try not to think right away about your upcoming day. Write down all of your dreams and images, as they can fade quickly if not recorded. Any distractions will cause the memory of your dream to fade. If you can't remember a full dream, record the last thing that was on your mind before awakening, even if you have only a vague memory of it.
>
> Source: Copyright © 2003 International Association for the Study of Dreams.

How can I learn to interpret my dreams?

The most important thing to keep in mind is that your dreams reflect your own underlying thoughts and feelings, and that the people, actions, settings, and emotions in your dreams are personal to you. Some dream experts theorize that there are typical or archetypal dreams and dream elements that persist across different persons, cultures, and times. Usually, however, the same image or symbol will have different meanings for different people. For example, an elephant in a dream can mean one thing to a zoo keeper and something quite different to a child whose favorite toy is a stuffed elephant. Therefore, books which give a specific meaning for a specific dream image or symbol (or "dream dictionaries") are not usually helpful. By thinking about what each dream element means to you or reminds you of, by looking for parallels between these associations and what is happening in your waking life, and by being patient and persistent, you can learn to understand your dreams. It can be helpful to keep a dream diary and reflect on many dreams over a long period of time to get the truest picture of your unique dream life. Many good books that can help you get started interpreting your dreams. [The International Association for the Study of Dreams (ASD) offers a list of suggestions online at http://www.asdreams.org/subidxedubookhelp.htm.]

What does it mean when I have the same dream over and over?

Recurrent dreams, which can continue for years, may be treated as any other dream. That is, one may look for parallels between the dream and the thoughts, feelings, behavior, and motives of the dreamer. Understanding the meaning of the recurrent dream sometimes can help the dreamer resolve an issue that he or she has been struggling with for years.

Is it normal to have nightmares?

Nightmares are very common among children and fairly common among adults. Often nightmares are caused by stress, traumatic experiences, emotional difficulties, drugs or medication, or illness. However, some people have frequent nightmares that seem unrelated to their waking lives. Recent studies suggest that these people tend to be more open, sensitive, trusting, and emotional than average. [ASD offers more information on nightmares online at http://www.asdreams.org/subidxedunightmares.htm.]

Is it true that if you dream that you die or that you hit bottom in a falling dream, you will in fact die in your sleep?

No, these beliefs are not true. Many people have dreamed that they died or hit bottom in a fall and they have lived to tell the tale. You can explore the meaning of these kinds of images just as you would explore any others that might occur in your dreams. However, if any aspect of your dreams worries or distresses you, talk to a professional mental health practitioner about your concerns.

Can dreams predict the future?

There are many examples of dreams that seemed to predict future events. Some may have been due to coincidence, faulty memory, or an unconscious tying together of known information. A few laboratory studies have been conducted of predictive dreams, as well as clairvoyant and telepathic dreams, but the results were varied, as these kinds of dreams are difficult to study in a laboratory setting.

Is it possible to control dreams?

You often can influence your dreams by giving yourself pre-sleep suggestions. Another method of influencing dreams is called lucid dreaming, in which you are aware you are dreaming while still asleep and in the dream. Sometimes people experience this type of dreaming spontaneously. It is often possible to learn how to increase lucid dreaming, and thereby increase your capacity to affect the course of the dream events as they unfold. Some things are easier than others to control, and indeed complete control is probably never possible. Some professional dream workers question the advisability of trying to control the dream, and encourage learning to enjoy and understand it instead.

Part Two

Sleep Habits

Chapter 6
How Much Sleep Do You Need?

Most teens need about 8½ to more than 9 hours of sleep each night. The right amount of sleep is essential for anyone who wants to do well on a test or play sports without tripping over their feet. Unfortunately, though, many teens don't get enough sleep.

Why aren't teens getting enough sleep?

Until recently, teens were often given a bad rap for staying up late, oversleeping for school, and falling asleep in class. But recent studies show that adolescent sleep patterns actually differ from those of adults or kids.

These studies show that during the teen years, the body's rhythm (sort of like an internal biological clock) is reset, telling a person to fall asleep later and wake up later. Unlike kids and adults, whose bodies tell them to go to sleep and wake up earlier, most teens' bodies tell them go to sleep late at night and sleep into the late morning. This change in the circadian rhythm seems to be due to the fact that the brain hormone is produced later at night for teens than it is for kids and adults. This can make it harder for teens to fall asleep early.

About This Chapter: This information was provided by TeensHealth, one of the largest resources online for medically reviewed health information written for parents, kids, and teens. For more articles like this one, visit www.TeensHealth.org, or www.KidsHealth.org. © 2004 The Nemours Foundation.

These changes in the body's circadian rhythm coincide with a time when we're busier than ever. For most teens, the pressure to do well in school is more intense than when they were kids, and it's harder to get by without studying hard. But teens also have other demands on their time—everything from sports and other extracurricular activities to fitting in a part-time job to save money for college.

Early start times in some schools also play a role in this sleep deficit. Teens who fall asleep after midnight may still have to get up early for school, meaning that they may only squeeze in 6 or 7 hours of sleep a night. A couple hours of missed sleep a night may not seem like a big deal, but can create a noticeable sleep deficit over time.

♣ It's A Fact!!
How much sleep is enough?

Every person is unique and so are our sleep needs. But in today's busy world, how much sleep should we be getting each night?

Research suggests that most healthy adults need seven to nine hours of sleep each night. Children and adolescents need even more sleep than adults. The following is a breakdown of the recommended number of hours of sleep people need by age (*including naps):

Infants
- 0 to 2 months: 10½ to 18 hours*
- 2–12 months: 14 to 15 hours*

Toddlers/Children
- 12–18 months: 13 to 15 hours*
- 18 months–3 years: 12 to 14 hours*
- 3–5 years: 11 to 13 hours*
- 5–12 years: 9 to 11 hours

Adolescents
- 8½ to 9½ hours

Why is sleep important?

This sleep deficit impacts everything from a person's ability to pay attention in class to his or her mood. Research shows that 20% of high school students fall asleep in class, and experts have been able to tie lost sleep to poorer grades. Lack of sleep also damages teens' ability to do their best in athletics.

Slowed responses and concentration from lack of sleep don't just affect school or sports performance, though. The fact that sleep deprivation slows reaction times can be life threatening for people who drive. The National Highway Safety Traffic Administration estimates that 1,500 people are killed every year in crashes caused by drivers between the ages of 15 and 24 who

Adults

• 7 to 9 hours

As children grow, they go through many changes, including changes in sleep. Children and teens, like adults, thrive on a regular sleep and wake schedule, even on the weekends. Sleep should follow a relaxing bedtime routine. The bedroom should be cool, dark, and quiet. Getting a good night's rest may become more difficult as they grow older due to increased responsibilities and activities, the impact of TV, computers, and caffeine or untreated sleep disorders. However, sleep is still a vital part of teens' performance, health, and overall quality of life, and should still be a priority.

So, how do teens measure how much sleep they need? If a teen has trouble staying alert during school, long drives, while reading a book, or in other quiet situations when sleepiness is often "unmasked," they probably are not getting enough quality sleep. Other signs of chronic sleep deprivation are irritability, difficulty concentrating or making decisions, loss of short-term memory, or becoming overly aggressive. In fact, sleep deprivation is often misdiagnosed as attention deficit hyperactivity disorder (ADHD).

Most sleep problems are treatable. If teens are having trouble getting the ZZZ's they need, it is important to see a doctor or other health professional.

Source: "How Much Sleep Is Enough?" © 2007 National Sleep Foundation (www.sleepfoundation.org). All rights reserved. Reprinted with permission.

are simply tired. (More than half of the people who cause crashes because they fall asleep at the wheel are under the age of 26.)

Lack of sleep has also been linked to emotional troubles, such as feelings of sadness and depression. Sleep helps keep us physically healthy, too, by slowing our body's systems enough to re-energize us after everyday activities.

How do I know if I'm getting enough?

Even if you think you're getting enough sleep, you may not be. Here are some of the signs that you may need more sleep:

- difficulty waking up in the morning

- inability to concentrate

- falling asleep during classes

- feelings of moodiness and even depression

How can I get more sleep?

Recently, some researchers, parents, and teachers have suggested that middle and high school classes begin later in the morning to accommodate teens' need for more sleep. Some schools have already implemented later start times. You and your friends, parents, and teachers can lobby for later start times at your school, but in the meantime you'll have to make your own adjustments.

Here are some things that may help you to sleep better:

- **Set a regular bedtime:** Going to bed at the same time each night signals to your body that it's time to sleep. Waking up at the same time every day can also help establish sleep patterns. So try to stick to your sleep schedule even on weekends. Don't go to sleep more than an hour later or wake up more than 2 to 3 hours later than you do during the week.

- **Exercise regularly:** Try not to exercise right before bed, though, as it can raise your body temperature and wake you up. Sleep experts believe that exercising 5 or 6 hours before bedtime (in late afternoon) may actually help a person sleep.

- **Avoid stimulants:** Don't drink beverages with caffeine, such as soda and coffee, after 4 P.M. Nicotine is also a stimulant, so quitting smoking may help you sleep better. And drinking alcohol in the evening can also cause a person to be restless and wake up during the night.

- **Relax your mind:** Avoid violent, scary, or action movies or television shows right before bed—anything that might set your mind and heart racing. Reading books with involved or active plots may also keep you from falling or staying asleep.

- **Unwind by keeping the lights low:** Light signals the brain that it's time to wake up. Staying away from bright lights (including computer screens), as well as meditating or listening to soothing music, can help your body relax.

- **Don't nap too much:** Naps of more than 30 minutes during the day may keep you from falling asleep later.

- **Avoid all-nighters:** Don't wait until the night before a big test to study. Cutting back on sleep the night before a test may mean you perform worse than you would if you'd studied less but got more sleep.

- **Create the right sleeping environment:** Studies show that people sleep best in a dark room that is slightly on the cool side. Close your blinds or curtains (and make sure they're heavy enough to block out light) and turn down the thermostat in your room (pile on extra blankets or wear PJs if you're cold). Lots of noise can be a sleep turnoff, too.

- **Wake up with bright light:** Bright light in the morning signals to your body that it's time to get going.

If you're drowsy, it's hard to look and feel your best. Schedule "sleep" as an item on your agenda to help you stay creative and healthy.

Chapter 7

Getting The Sleep You Need

Sleep is one of the body's most mysterious processes. The idea of sleeping well conjures up restful images of fluffy pillows, comfortable blankets, and minimal activity. However, many people find sleep elusive. And the more we worry about our insomnia, the worse our sleep problems get. Use this chapter for "sleep literacy" to help you to get the sleep you need.

What happens when we sleep?

Sleep is a periodic state of rest during which consciousness of the world is interrupted. Additionally, sleep is marked by:

- decreased movement of the skeletal muscles;

- a relaxed posture, usually lying down;

- reduced response to stimulation, such as sounds and touch;

- slowed-down metabolism; and

- complex and active brain wave patterns.

What are the stages of sleep in the sleep cycle?

Sleep is divided into two types: REM (rapid eye movement) sleep and NREM (non-REM) sleep. REM sleep is when we dream. NREM sleep is further divided into four stages. A typical night of sleep follows this pattern:

- **Stage 1 (Drowsiness):** When you first fall asleep, you are in Stage 1 sleep (drowsiness). Stage 1 lasts just five or ten minutes. Eyes move slowly under the eyelids, and muscle activity slows down. You are easily awakened during Stage 1 sleep.

- **Stage 2 (Light Sleep):** Next, you go into Stage 2 sleep (light sleep). In Stage 2, eye movements stop, heart rate slows, and body temperature decreases.

- **Stages 3 And 4 (Deep Sleep):** Then you enter Stages 3 and 4 (deep sleep). During stages 3 and 4, you are difficult to awaken. People who are awakened during deep sleep do not adjust immediately and often feel groggy and disoriented for several minutes after they wake up. Children may experience bedwetting, night terrors, or sleepwalking during deep sleep.

- **REM Sleep:** At about 70 to 90 minutes into your sleep cycle, you enter REM sleep. You usually have three to five REM episodes per night. Your eyes jerk rapidly in various directions under your eyelids, thus the name rapid eye movement (REM) sleep.

The first sleep cycles each night contain relatively short REM periods and long periods of deep sleep. As the night progresses, REM sleep periods increase in length while deep sleep decreases. By morning, people spend nearly all their sleep time in stages 1, 2, and REM.

What happens during the REM sleep stage?

During REM sleep, you dream actively, but your limb muscles are immobile. Your breathing is rapid, irregular, and shallow. Your heart rate increases, your blood pressure rises, males may have penile erections, and females may have clitoral enlargement. Your brain is at least as active during REM sleep as it is when you are awake.

Because your major muscles do not move during REM sleep, you will not act out your dreams. (Sleepwalking occurs during NREM sleep.)

If our REM sleep is disrupted one night, our bodies don't follow the normal sleep cycle progression the next time we doze off. Instead, we often slip directly into REM sleep and go through extended periods of REM until we "catch up" on this stage of sleep.

Infants spend about 50 percent of their sleep time in REM sleep; after infancy, you spend fifteen to twenty percent of your sleep time in REM sleep.

♣ It's A Fact!!

Why does my body jerk before I fall asleep?

You're just about to drift off into a deep sleep when suddenly you feel like you're falling or rolling downhill on a roller coaster. Then your body jerks suddenly and you're awake. Weird! What's going on?

This body movement, also known as a sleep start, is what doctors and scientists call a hypnic (say: hip-nik) or myoclonic (say: my-uh-klah-nik) jerk.

These jerks usually occur before you enter the deeper stages of sleep and are completely normal. Doctors and scientists aren't really sure why they happen, but they have a few theories.

One theory is that your brain misunderstands the sensation of your muscles relaxing as you drift off to sleep. It's normal for the muscles to relax, but the brain gets confused, and, for a minute, thinks you're falling. In response, the brain causes your muscles to tense up so you "catch yourself" before you fall down.

These jerks can wake a person up, or the person might just keep on sleeping. They're nothing to worry about, so if one of them wakes you up, snuggle back under your quilt, and try to catch some more ZZZs.

Source: This information was provided by KidsHealth, one of the largest resources online for medically reviewed health information written for parents, kids, and teens. For more articles like this one, visit www.KidsHealth.org, or www.TeensHealth.org. © 2004 The Nemours Foundation.

Why do we need sleep?

Sleep helps you to restore and rejuvenate many body functions:

- **Memory And Learning:** Sleep seems to organize memories, as well as help you to recover memories. After you learn something new, sleep may solidify the learning in your brain.

- **Mood Enhancement And Social Behaviors:** The parts of the brain that control emotions, decision-making, and social interactions slow down dramatically during sleep, allowing optimal performance when awake. REM sleep seems especially important for a good mood during the day. Tired people are often cranky and easily frustrated.

- **Nervous System:** Some sleep experts suggest that neurons used during the day repair themselves during sleep. When we experience sleep deprivation, neurons are unable to perform effectively, and the nervous system is impaired.

- **Immune System:** Without adequate sleep, the immune system becomes weak, and the body becomes more vulnerable to infection and disease.

- **Growth And Development:** Growth hormones are released during sleep, and sleep is vital to proper physical and mental development.

What are some of the effects of sleep deprivation?

Lack of sleep, and especially a chronic lack of sleep, is associated with the following characteristics:

- Poor decision-making, poor judgment, increased risk-taking
- Poor performance in school, on the job, and in sports
- Impaired driving performance and more car accidents
- Increased incidence of obesity, diabetes, illness in general, high blood pressure, and heart disease
- Impaired memory, concentration, and ability to learn
- Physical impairment, poor coordination, delayed reaction time
- Anxiety, depression, and other emotional problems

- Magnification of the effects of alcohol on the body

- Exacerbation of the symptoms of attention deficit hyperactivity disorder (ADHD), such as impulse control, irritability, and lack of concentration

- Getting less than six hours of sleep per night can affect coordination, reaction time, and judgment. A study reported in *Occupational and Environmental Medicine* (September 2000) comparing the effects of sleep deprivation and alcohol found that "people who drive after being awake for 17 to 19 hours performed worse than those with a blood alcohol level of .05 percent [the legal limit for drunkenness in most European countries]."

How much sleep do we need?

The amount of sleep that you need depends on a number of factors, including:

- your genetic make-up,

- the amount of exercise you get,

- what you do during your waking hours,

- your age,

- whether you are still growing, and

- the quality of your sleep.

Table 7.1 lists some guidelines on how much sleep people might need.

> ✔ **Quick Tip**
>
> **A rule of thumb:** If you wake up feeling refreshed, and you don't feel sleepy during the day, you are getting enough sleep. If you have an occasional night of poor sleep, you probably will need to sleep more the next night to make up for it.
>
> Source: © 2007 Helpguide.org.

What are the signs of sleep deprivation and how can I tell if I have a sleep debt?

Some of the signs of sleep deprivation include:

- difficulty waking up in the morning,

- lack of concentration,

- falling asleep during work or class, and

- feelings of moodiness, irritability, depression, or anxiety.

If you are tired or drowsy during the day, you probably haven't gotten enough sleep, and you have a "sleep debt." A sleep debt can be from one night's poor sleep or the accumulation of many days of not enough sleep.

You can make up for a sleep debt with extra sleep, but a chronic sleep debt can have serious long-term effects, including immune system problems, metabolic changes that can lead to obesity, and hyperactivity.

The Epworth Sleepiness Scale is a standard simple test to determine your sleep debt. You can try an online test of sleep debt and get an instant tally of your level of sleepiness at http://www.smmc.com/Epworth-Sleepiness-Scale .105.0.html.

Table 7.1. Typical Sleep Needs

Group	Amount of Sleep Needed
Infants	About 16 hours per day of sleep
Babies and toddlers	From 6 months to 3 years: between 10 and 14 hours per day. Young children generally get their sleep from a combination of nighttime sleep and naps.
Children	Ages 3 to 6: between 10 and 12 hours of sleep Ages 6 to 9: about 10 hours of sleep Ages 9 to 12: about 9 hours of sleep
Teenagers	About 9 hours of sleep per night. Teens have trouble getting enough sleep not only because of their busy schedules, but also because they are biologically programmed to want to stay up later and sleep later in the morning, which usually doesn't mesh with school schedules.
Adults	For most adults, 7 to 8 hours a night appears to be the best amount of sleep, although some people may need as few as 5 hours or as many as 10 hours of sleep each night.
Older adults	Current thought is that older adults need as much, if not more, sleep than middle-aged adults. Taking a midday nap may help.
Pregnant women	During pregnancy, women may need a few more hours of sleep per night.

How can I use a sleep diary to assess my sleep patterns and sleep habits?

Learn about your sleep patterns and habits ("sleep hygiene") by keeping a daily sleep diary. You can see Helpguide's sample sleep diary online at http://www.helpguide.org/life/sleep_diary.pdf, or make up your own sleep log and include:

- the times you went to bed and woke up,

- total sleep hours,

- quality of your sleep,

- the times that you were awake during the night and what you did (for example, stayed in bed with eyes closed, or got up, had a glass of milk, and meditated),

- amount of caffeine, alcohol, or nicotine you consumed and times of consumption,

- types of food and drink before bed and times of consumption,

- your feelings (happiness, sadness, stress, anxiety), and

- any drugs or medications taken, amounts taken, and times of consumption.

What are some tips to help with my sleeping?

Establishing a consistent sleep routine is one of the most important ways to ensure a good night's sleep. Following are a few pre-sleep routines that might work for you:

- **Keep a consistent sleep schedule:** Try not to vary the hours when you go to bed and when you wake up, even on weekends. A consistent sleep schedule trains your body to go to sleep and wake up at set times.

- **Develop relaxing bedtime rituals:** Listen to soft music, sip a cup of herbal tea or warm milk, or meditate.

- **Limit your intake of caffeine, and nicotine:** Insomniacs may be hypersensitive to caffeine, and even small amounts may affect your sleep. Nicotine is a stimulant and deters sleep. In addition, teens should not consume any alcohol, and adults need to limit intake of alcohol. Although people may think that alcohol helps them fall asleep, it interferes with deep sleep.

- **Limit your intake of food right before bed:** Eat no more than a light snack within the last two to three hours before bed. A large, heavy meal can interfere with your sleep.

- **Reserve your bedroom for sleep:** Move the television to another room. Don't initiate important relationship discussions or have arguments in the bedroom.

- **Clear your mind of anxious thoughts:** Before you retire to the bedroom, write down anything you need to remember for tomorrow so that you don't have to worry as you go to bed.

- **Exercise early in the day:** Exercising late in the day can make you feel too awake to sleep.

- **Take a hot bath to induce a drop in your body temperature:** The onset of sleep is correlated with a drop in body temperature. If you have difficulty going to sleep, take a hot bath 90 minutes before bedtime so that your temperature has to decrease afterwards.

Can sleep medications and sleeping pills help me to sleep better?

Often, people turn to sleeping pills to help them sleep. However, using sleep medications to treat insomnia is risky for many reasons:

- Sleep medications do not treat the root cause of your sleep problem and can ultimately exacerbate your insomnia.

- Some prescription sleeping pills are addictive, and you may condition yourself to rely on them for sleep.

- You can develop a tolerance for sleep medications and require larger and larger doses to feel their effects.

- The side-effects of sleeping pills can be significant.

- Sleep medications interfere with deep sleep, and their sedative effects can extend into daytime activities as well.

Chapter 8

The Sleep Environment

Does that drip, drip, drip of the faucet keep you up at night? Do you need to keep your fan running because "white noise" helps you sleep? Have you ever tossed and turned because you were too hot, or too cold? What about the barking dog or cat that jumps onto your bed—have they ever disrupted your ZZZs? Most of us recognize that the sleep environment can greatly affect how (and if) we sleep, but are you doing everything you can to make your bedroom a sleep haven? Learn about the do's and don'ts of the sleep environment and then get tips for making your bedroom more sleep-friendly.

Noise

Noises at levels as low as 40 decibels or as high as 70 decibels generally keep us awake. That means that a dripping faucet can steal your sleep, as well as the next door neighbor's blaring stereo. But the absence or presence of a familiar noise can have as great an impact on your sleep as out-of-the-ordinary noises—studies show that sirens and traffic noise from a city street can actually become soothing to longtime city sleepers (they will cringe at the thought of sleeping in the serene desert or mountain climate) just as the absence of the tick, tick, tick of your favorite clock while you try to sleep at a hotel can become a sleep stealer.

What To Do: Try to block out unwanted sounds with earplugs or use "white noise" such as a fan or an air conditioner. Take your favorite clock with you when you travel in order to recreate familiar sounds that help you sleep (as long as they won't keep your neighbors awake).

Temperature

In most cases, temperatures above 75 degrees Fahrenheit and below 54 degrees will disrupt sleep, but even sleep researchers fail to agree on the ideal temperature for sleep. The point at which sleep is interrupted due to temperature or climate conditions varies from person to person and can be affected by bed clothes and bedding materials selected by the sleeper. In general, most sleep scientists believe that a slightly cool room contributes to good sleep. That's because it mimics what occurs inside the body when the body's internal temperature drops during the night to its lowest level. (For good sleepers, this occurs about four hours after they begin sleeping.)

What To Do: In general, sleep scientists recommend keeping your room slightly cool—but achieving the ideal temperature isn't always simple. What do you do if you and your partner disagree about room temperature? Turning the thermostat down at night in cold weather saves on fuel bills and sets the stage for sleep. Blankets, comforters, or electric blankets can lock in heat without feeling too heavy or confining. Or the heat-seeking partner might dress in warmer bedclothes while the warmer partner might opt not to wear sleep clothes or bed covering. In summer, a room that's too hot can also be disruptive. In fact, research suggests that a hot sleeping environment leads to more wake time and lighter sleep at night, while awakenings multiply. An air conditioner or fan can help, and a humidifier can provide relief if you're suffering from a sore throat or dryness in your nose.

Light

Much of our sleep patterns—feeling sleepy at night and awake during the day—are regulated by light and darkness. Light—strong light, like bright outdoor light (which is brighter than indoor light even on cloudy days)—is the most powerful regulator of our biological clock. The biological clock influences when we feel sleepy and when we feel alert. As a result, finding the balance of light and darkness exposure is important. Bright light helps to keep you awake during the day, but during sleep, bright lights can be disturbing.

What To Do: Make sure to expose yourself to enough bright light during the day. Find time for sunlight, or purchase a lightbox or light visor to supplement your exposure to light. At bedtime, think dark: a dark bedroom contributes to better sleep. Try light-blocking curtains, drapes, or an eye mask. If you find yourself waking earlier than you'd like, try increasing your exposure to bright light in the evening. It may delay sleep onset but as little as one to two hours of evening bright light exposure may help you sleep longer in the morning. Also, make sure to avoid light if you wake up in the middle of the night to go to the bathroom. Minimize light by using a low illumination night light.

Sleeping Surface

For the most part, we know people sleep better when horizontal and not cramped by space. Not much research has been done to understand the sleeping surface, but it is clear that it plays a role in getting a good night's sleep. For example, tossing and turning on a lumpy 20-year-old mattress that doesn't provide support for your back or neck can impede you from getting the sleep you need and make you very sleepy (and stiff) the next day. Mattress experts say that too often consumers believe that ultra-firm mattresses are good for them, but research on patients with back pain found this was not true and a more supple, comforting mattress may lead to better sleep.

> ♣ **It's A Fact!!**
> One study found that synthetic pillows had as much as five times more dust-mite fecal matter than feather pillows (feather pillows have thick casing to keeps feathers in).

Also, know your pillow: research shows that pillows house thousands of fungal spores which can trigger allergies and compromise a weakened immune system. The research shows that synthetic pillows held a greater amount of bacteria than feather pillows. So, not only can a pillow affect your posture and quality of sleep, but it can also affect your allergies or asthma and make it very difficult to get a good night's rest.

What To Do: Give yourself enough space to sleep. If you share a bed with a partner, make sure it is large enough to give both of you room to move around. Replace an old mattress with a new one, and choose a pillow and mattress that fits you best (soft, firm, thick, thin?) and will be comfortable throughout the whole night. Consumer Reports recently found that consumers who spent 15 minutes or more testing each mattress at the store were more likely to be happy with their purchase. Also, consider encasing your pillow in a plastic cover under your pillowcase to keep dust-mites from interfering with your sleep and allergy or asthma symptoms.

Other Factors

Bed Partners: Bed partners with sleep disorders can negatively impact your sleep. Have you ever been kept awake by your partner's snoring? Or been jolted out of a sound sleep by your partner's restless movements? If so, you're not alone. According to the National Sleep Foundation's (NSF) 2005 Sleep in America poll, 67% of respondents reported that their partner snores, 27% said their intimate relationship was affected because they were too sleepy, and 38% said they have had problems in their relationship due to their partner's sleep disorder.

What To Do: Start off by talking to your partner about the problem. If he/she has not sought treatment for a potential sleep disorder, encourage them to see a doctor. Consider ear plugs if snoring prevents your sleep. Try to create a sleeping arrangement that is comfortable for both you and your partner. Keep the lines of communication open.

> ✔ **Quick Tip**
>
> TVs, computers, and work in the bedroom are sleep stealing culprits. National Sleep Foundation's 2005 Sleep in America poll found that 87% of respondents watched TV within an hour of going to bed at least a few nights a week. Doing work, watching TV, and using the computer, both close to bedtime and especially in the bedroom, hinders quality sleep. Violent shows, news reports, and stories before bedtime can be agitating. The sleep environment should be used only for sleep and sex.
>
> **What To Do:** Avoid highly engaging activities such as watching dramatic TV or doing work close to bedtime. Keep the TV and computer out of your bedroom! Make your bedroom a place that is centered around sleep.

Pets: Cats and dogs can be cuddly in bed, but they may be interfering with your sleep. Anyone who has slept with another person in their bed knows that sharing a sleeping space can be disruptive, but when your four-legged friend gets added to the mix, it becomes even more complicated. While a pet can make your sleep environment more comfortable, it is not mindful of whether it is interfering with your sleep.

What To Do: Think about providing your dog or cat with a bed in your bedroom, instead of sharing your bed. Well-rested pet owners will have more energy and love to give to their pets.

Chapter 9

Sleeping Tips

Falling asleep isn't as easy as falling off a log. To fall asleep and sleep well, try these tips:

- Go to sleep and wake up at the same time every day, even on the weekends.

- Our brains are built to sleep when it's dark. Changes in light help us know when to sleep and when to be awake. (You ever notice how it's harder to wake up on dreary, rainy days?) When it's dark, your brain makes a chemical called melatonin that makes you sleepy. When you're in the light, your brain shuts off the melatonin. Light wakes you up, so your room should be dark when you sleep. Even the light from a television or computer screen can make it harder to fall asleep. A dim nightlight is okay. You should get into bright light as soon as possible in the morning to help "turn off" melatonin and wake you up! Turn on the light, pull back the curtains, or go outside to check the temperature.

- Know your body's daily rhythm. For example, if you get sleepy early in the afternoon, and you have class, try to move around right before. That'll wake you up so you're not snoozing. If you're more of a night person, schedule exercise after school, not when you wake up in the morning.

About This Chapter: "Expert's Opinion: Sleeping Tips," and "Questions Answered," BAM! Body and Mind (www.bam.gov), 2005.

- Don't drink coffee, sodas with caffeine, or drinks and snacks with lots of sugar. They can make you feel too wired, and caffeine can make it hard to fall asleep even hours later.

- Being active can help you sleep better, but don't exercise less than 3 hours before bed—getting your blood pumping like that can make it hard to fall asleep. Take a cue from the sun and start gearing down when the sun sets.

- Relax before going to bed. Avoid anything that requires serious concentration, like heavy reading or studying, within an hour of going to bed.

♣ It's A Fact!! Feeling Sleepy? Here's Why!

- Many teens need at least 9 hours of sleep per night. More than younger kids, and more than adults. But most teens get less than 6.5 hours of sleep. If "most teens" is you, you're probably sleepy most of the time.

- When kids hit puberty, their internal clocks change: that's why teens just naturally want to go to bed late and sleep late in the morning!

- Teenagers have more responsibilities than younger kids. And, between school, homework, jobs, sports and a social life, it is difficult for them to get enough sleep.

Source: "Awake at the Wheel," National Heart, Lung, and Blood Institute, 1997.

- Use your bed only for sleeping—don't do homework or talk on the phone when you're in bed. That way, your body starts to know that once you're in bed, it's time for sleep.

Questions Answered

The night before a big test, should I stay up as late as possible so I can study more?

If you've got a ton to learn, it's best to study a little bit every day, rather than cramming the night before the test. You're better off getting a good night's sleep before a test than spending all night studying. That's because sleep has a big role in memory. Sleep helps everything you've studied "set" in your mind, so you can remember it later. It's like pressing "save" after working

on a computer. Getting enough sleep also helps you pay attention and concentrate the next day. Make sure you leave yourself enough time the night
before the test so you can review what you need to, and still get to bed at
your normal time.

If you feel sluggish, drinking a soda with caffeine or lots of sugar can help you catch up and feel more energetic, right?

While caffeine and sugar might pick you up short term, they'll leave you
even more drained than before. Drinking caffeine can affect your sleep, even
hours later. It can create a vicious cycle: you feel drained, so you down a soda,
but then that night you can't sleep well, so you feel drained the next day, so
you have another soda, and on and on. The ups and downs can make you feel
like you're on a roller coaster; and the longer you stay on, the lower the lows
are, and the more caffeine or sugar it takes to get you back up. Also, caffeine
and sugar don't have any of the other good effects of sleep, like improving
memory and concentration, or helping your body regulate growth and tons
of other stuff. It's much better to get enough sleep. Set a regular schedule for
waking up and going to bed. Calm down in the last hour before bedtime,
and make your bedroom quiet, cool, and dark.

How do I know how much sleep I need?

Kids who are 7 to 11 years old need at least 9 hours of sleep a night. But
everyone's different—the surefire way to tell if you've gotten enough sleep is
if you wake up feeling refreshed. You don't need to bounce out of bed, but if
you wake up dragging and willing to sell your kid sister for an extra half-
hour, you should hit the sheets earlier tonight.

✔ Quick Tip
If you wake up without your alarm
clock, that's a sign you've slept enough.

Source: "Questions Answered," BAM! Body and Mind, 2005.

I have such a hard time getting up in the morning—this never used to happen. What's going on?

Everyone has an internal clock that controls when you get sleepy and when you're wide awake. There's a big shift in your internal clock when you go through puberty—it gets later, which means as you get older, you might not be able to fall asleep until 11 p.m., and you might want to sleep through the morning.

You might want to go to bed late and sleep in on the weekends, but keeping this schedule means it can be tough to get up on Monday morning.

The best way to cope with this is to keep a consistent schedule—go to bed and wake up at the same time every day, weekend or weekday.

Sometimes I toss and turn for a long time before I fall asleep. What should I do to fall asleep faster?

Have no fear! There are things you can do to calm down before bedtime.

- Relax for an hour at least before bedtime. This isn't the time for push-ups or that hilarious movie that makes you laugh 'til your side hurts.

- Your body temperature drops at night, which is one signal to your body to get sleep. Taking a warm bath before bedtime is one trick to fool your body—when your temperature drops after the bath, it will signal bedtime.

- Don't eat a heavy meal within a few hours of bedtime. All the blood will go to your stomach to digest it and keep you up.

- You can have a light snack before bed. Try a cup of warm milk—it's known for bringing on the ZZZs.

> ### ♣ It's A Fact!!
> There's a nap-friendly substance in milk called tryptophan (it's also in turkey, which may be why you want to take a nap after Thanksgiving dinner). Also, like having a warm bath, drinking warm milk will raise your temperature a little bit, and then it will drop back to normal. The drop in temperature can trigger sleep because it reminds your body of falling asleep (when your body temperature drops naturally).
>
> Source: "Questions Answered," BAM! Body and Mind, 2005.

- Try not to have any caffeine, and if you do, don't have any after lunch. Same goes for sugary drinks or treats. Sugar and caffeine give you a burst of energy that'll make you too wired to snooze.

- If your worries are keeping you up, write them down. Putting them down on paper helps keep them from rattling around in your head.

- Try and make your room as much like a cave as possible—quiet, cool, dark, and peaceful. Turn off the radio, TV, or anything noisy, and draw the shades.

- When you get in bed, turn your clock away from your bed and take deep breaths.

- Staying in bed when you can't fall asleep can be stressful. If you're tossing and turning, get out of bed and do something calm, like reading in dim light, until you feel tired again. Then go back to bed.

Over the long run, you can improve your sleep by:

- Trying to go to bed and wake up at the same time every day.

- Being active at least a few hours before bedtime. That'll use up energy during the day, and give you enough time to calm down before hitting the sack.

- Training your brain so that when it sees your bed, it thinks, "sleep." Do homework and chat on the phone somewhere else.

Chapter 10

What To Do If You Can't Sleep

Sometimes going to sleep can seem boring. There's so much more you want to do. But if you've ever had too little sleep, you know that you don't feel very well when you're not rested. Some kids have trouble falling to sleep. Let's talk about what to do if that happens to you.

Bedtime Fears

For kids, feeling scared or worried at bedtime is one of the main reasons for having trouble falling asleep. A kid might be afraid of the dark or might not like being alone. If a kid has a good imagination, he or she might hear noises at night and fear the worst—when it's just the family cat walking down the hall.

As you get older, these fears usually fade. Until they do, make sure your room makes you feel relaxed and peaceful. Look around your room from your bed. Are there things you can see from bed that make you feel good? If not, add some. Display some family photos or other pictures that make you happy. You might even create a mobile to hang over your bed.

About This Chapter: This information was provided by KidsHealth, one of the largest resources online for medically reviewed health information written for parents, kids, and teens. For more articles like this one, visit www.KidsHealth.org, or www.TeensHealth.org. © 2005 The Nemours Foundation.

Nightmares

Have you been having any nightmares lately? Sometimes it's hard to fall asleep when you're afraid of having a scary dream that feels way too real. If the fear of nightmares is keeping you awake, try talking to your mom or dad. Sometimes talking about the nightmares (and even drawing a picture of them) can help you stop having them.

By the way, kids have many more bad dreams when they watch scary or violent TV shows or movies or read scary books or stories before bedtime. Instead of doing those kinds of things, try thinking good thoughts before bed. Imagine a favorite place or activity or think of all the people who care about you. Reading a peaceful book before bed (your parent can read to you, or you can read to yourself) or playing soothing music can help you have sweet dreams.

Worry And Stress

Insomnia also can happen when you're worried about things. It's easy to feel stressed when you have tests at school, after-school activities, team sports, and chores around the house. If you're starting to feel overwhelmed—like it's all just too much—speak up. Your mom or dad can help you put some balance in your schedule. It may mean cutting out some activities so you have more free time.

Big Changes

A major change in your life or daily routine can easily cause sleep problems. Changes like divorce, death, illness, or moving to a new town can affect your ability to sleep through the night. During a difficult time, it helps if you feel safe. Try bringing a comforting object to bed with you, like a blanket a relative made for you or a favorite stuffed animal. It might take a while to feel better, so talk with your mom or dad about what's bothering you. Even if the problem can't be solved, just talking it out can help you sleep easier.

Feeling Uncomfortable

If you feel too hot, too cold, hungry, or crowded, you won't get to sleep like you should. Prevent this by creating sleep-friendly bedtime space:

♣ It's A Fact!!
Tired, But Wired

Both kids and adults get insomnia, but it doesn't affect them the same way. Kids who are deprived of sleep often feel hyper—like they're bouncing off the walls. Adults, on the other hand, feel sluggish and tired.

• Make sure your bed is ready for sleep and relaxing—not so jammed with toys and stuffed animals that there's no room for you.

• Turn on a fan if you're warm or pull on some socks if you're cold.

• Have a regular bedtime routine that includes a light snack if you often feel hungry when it's time to turn in.

Getting Help For Sleep Woes

Most of the time, talking with your parent is all you need to do to handle a sleep problem. Your mom or dad can help you improve your bedtime routine and help you be patient while you develop new sleep habits. But if a kid has really tough sleep problems, he or she might need extra help.

That could mean talking to a counselor or psychologist about stress or sadness the kid is feeling. If the kid's not really worried about anything, he or she could have a sleep problem. In this case, the answer might be to see a doctor who's a specialist in sleep. Some hospitals even have sleep labs, where patients come in and go to sleep so doctors can monitor their sleep and see what might be wrong.

Sleep Tips

Because so many people get insomnia, there has been a lot of research done on how to beat it. Lucky for you, right? Not all of these tips work for everyone, but one or two might help you.

• Write in a journal before you go to bed. This practice clears your mind so you won't have all those thoughts crowding your brain when you're trying to sleep.

• Sleep in a dark, comfortable room. Light signals your body that it's time to be awake, so you want to avoid it at night. But if you are really afraid of the dark, it's OK to try a dim night-light. And being hot and sweaty or shivering from the cold can easily keep you up.

- Don't sleep with a pet. This can be a tough habit to break, but your lovable dog or cat could be keeping you awake. As your pet cozies up to you or makes noise, it could wake you from a peaceful sleep. Try sleeping without your pet for a couple nights to see if you sleep better that way.

- Don't drink any caffeinated beverages (like soda or iced tea) after about 3:00 in the afternoon. Caffeine is a stimulant and might keep you awake.

- Don't exercise at night. Keep your exercise to earlier in the day—never within a couple hours of when you go to sleep.

- Once you're lying in bed, try a peaceful mind exercise. For instance, count backward from 100 with your eyes closed. By the time you get to 10 (yawn) we hope you'll feel very sleepy. And by 5, we hope you'll feel yourself drifting off ... 3, 2, 1, ZZZZZZZZZZZZZZZ.

Chapter 11

Caffeine: What You Should Know

It's 11:00 P.M. and you've already had a full day of school and after-school activities. You're tired and you know you could use some sleep, but you still haven't finished your homework or watched the movie that's due back tomorrow. So instead of catching a few ZZZs, you reach for the remote—and the caffeine.

What Is Caffeine?

Caffeine is a drug that is naturally produced in the leaves and seeds of many plants. It's also produced artificially and added to certain foods. It's part of the same group of drugs sometimes used to treat asthma.

Caffeine is defined as a drug because it stimulates the central nervous system, causing increased heart rate and alertness. Most people who are sensitive to caffeine experience a temporary increase in energy and elevation in mood.

Caffeine is in tea leaves, coffee beans, chocolate, many soft drinks, pain relievers, and other over-the-counter pills. In its natural form, caffeine tastes very bitter. But most caffeinated drinks have gone through enough processing to camouflage the bitter taste. Most teens get the majority of their caffeine intake through soft drinks, which can also have added sugar and artificial flavors.

About This Chapter: This information, from "Caffeine," was provided by TeensHealth, one of the largest resources online for medically reviewed health information written for parents, kids, and teens. For more articles like this one, visit www.TeensHealth.org, or www.KidsHealth.org. © 2004 The Nemours Foundation.

Got The Jitters?

If taken in moderate amounts (like a single can of soda or cup of coffee), many people feel that caffeine increases their mental alertness. Higher doses of caffeine can cause anxiety, dizziness, headaches, and the jitters and can interfere with normal sleep, though. And very high doses of caffeine—like taking a whole box of alertness pills—would be harmful to the body.

Caffeine is addictive and may cause withdrawal symptoms for those who abruptly stop consuming it. These include severe headaches, muscle aches, temporary depression, and irritability. Although scientists once worried that caffeine could stunt growth, this concern is not supported by research.

Caffeine sensitivity refers to the amount of caffeine that will produce an effect in someone. This amount varies from person to person. On average, the smaller the person, the less caffeine necessary to produce side effects. However, caffeine sensitivity is most affected by the amount of daily caffeine use. People who regularly drink beverages containing caffeine soon develop a reduced sensitivity to caffeine. This means they require higher doses of caffeine to achieve the same effects as someone who doesn't drink caffeinated drinks every day. In short, the more caffeine you take in, the more caffeine you'll need to feel the same effects.

Although you may think you're getting plenty of liquids when you drink caffeinated beverages, caffeine works against the body in two ways: It has a mild dehydrating effect because it increases the need to urinate. And large amounts of caffeine may cause the body to lose calcium and potassium, causing sore muscles and delayed recovery times after exercise.

Caffeine has health risks for certain users. Small children are more sensitive to caffeine because they have not been exposed to it as much as older children or adults. Pregnant women or nursing mothers should consider decreasing their caffeine intake, although in small or moderate amounts

♣ It's A Fact!!

Caffeine moves through the body within a few hours after it's consumed and is then passed through the urine. It's not stored in the body, but you may feel its effects for up to 6 hours if you're sensitive to it.

there is no evidence that it causes a problem for the baby. Caffeine can aggravate heart problems or nervous disorders, and some teens may not be aware that they're at risk.

Moderation Is The Key

Although the effects of caffeine vary from one person to the next, doctors recommend that people should consume no more than about 100 milligrams (mg) of caffeine daily. That might sound like a lot, but one espresso contains about 100 milligrams of caffeine. Table 11.1 includes common caffeinated products and the amounts of caffeine they contain.

Table 11.1. The Amount Of Caffeine In Common Caffeinated Products

Drink/Food	Amt. of Drink/Food	Amt. of Caffeine
Jolt soft drink	12 ounces	71.2 mg
Mountain Dew	12 ounces	55.0 mg
Coca-Cola	12 ounces	34.0 mg
Diet Coke	12 ounces	45.0 mg
Pepsi	12 ounces	38.0 mg
7-Up	12 ounces	0 mg
Brewed coffee (drip method)	5 ounces	115 mg*
Iced tea	12 ounces	70 mg*
Dark chocolate	1 ounce	20 mg*
Milk chocolate	1 ounce	6 mg*
Cocoa beverage	5 ounces	4 mg*
Chocolate milk beverage	8 ounces	5 mg*
Cold relief medication	1 tablet	30 mg*
Vivarin	1 tablet	200 mg

* denotes average amount of caffeine

Source: U.S. Food and Drug Administration and National Soft Drink Association.

Cutting Back

If you're taking in too much caffeine, you may want to cut back. Kicking the caffeine habit is never easy, and the best way is to cut back slowly. Otherwise you could get headaches and feel achy, depressed, or lousy.

Try cutting your intake by substituting noncaffeinated drinks for caffeinated sodas and coffee. Examples include water, caffeine-free sodas, and caffeine-free teas. Keep track of how many caffeinated drinks you have each day, and substitute one drink per week with a caffeine-free alternative until you've gotten below the 100-milligram mark.

✔ Quick Tip

As you cut back on the amount of caffeine you consume, you may find yourself feeling tired. Your best bet is to hit the sack, not the sodas: It's just your body's way of telling you it needs more rest. Your energy levels will return to normal in a few days.

Chapter 12

Anxiety Can Affect Sleep

It's 1:15 A.M. and Morgan can't sleep because she's worried about the math test she has in the morning. Actually, it seems like she worries about almost everything these days. What if she oversleeps and misses the bus? Did she remember to put pads in her bag in case she gets her period tomorrow? Why hadn't Maya called her back tonight? How will she work at the store all day Saturday and still have time to write the paper that's due on Monday? It's another 45 minutes before Morgan is finally able to drift off.

It's completely normal to worry about your hectic, complicated life, but if the worries become overwhelming, you may feel that they're running your life. If you spend an excessive amount of time feeling anxious or you have difficulty sleeping because of your anxiety, pay attention to your thoughts and feelings. They may be symptoms of an anxiety problem or disorder.

What Is Anxiety?

Anxiety is a natural part of life, and most of us experience it from time to time. The word "anxiety" usually refers to worry, concern, stress, or nervousness. For most teens, anxiety is limited to particular situations such as tests, important dates (like the prom), or driving lessons.

About This Chapter: This information, from "All About Anxiety," was provided by TeensHealth, one of the largest resources online for medically reviewed health information written for parents, kids, and teens. For more articles like this one, visit www.TeensHealth.org, or www.KidsHealth.org. © 2004 The Nemours Foundation.

But for some teens, anxiety is a constant factor in their lives. When a person has an anxiety disorder, it interferes with their ability to function normally on a daily basis. Anxiety disorders can cause teens to suffer from intense, long-lasting fear or worry, in addition to other symptoms.

♣ **It's A Fact!!**
Feeling anxious can sometimes be a good thing. Anxiety can actually help you by motivating you to prepare for a big test or by keeping you on your toes in potentially dangerous situations. Occasional anxiety isn't something to be concerned about.

Understanding Anxiety Disorders

Anxiety disorders are conditions that involve unrealistic fear and worry. Anxiety disorders are very common—it is estimated that that they affect about 13% of the U.S. population. Anxiety disorders affect people of all ages, including kids and teens.

A teen who has an anxiety disorder isn't "crazy," and certainly isn't alone. Many teens have anxiety disorders, and have feelings of fear, worry, panic, or intense stress that can sometimes make it hard to get through the day. Anxiety can also interfere with things as basic as sleep, concentration, and appetite, not to mention the ability to enjoy life and relax. The good news is that anxiety disorders are very treatable.

There are several types of anxiety disorders that can affect teens. They include:

Generalized anxiety disorder, or GAD, for example, refers to constant, intense worry and stress about a variety of everyday things or situations. Teens with GAD may worry about school, health or safety of family members, the future, and whether they'll become ill or injured. They may always think of the worst that could happen. Along with the worry and dread, they may have physical symptoms, too, such as chest pain, headache, tiredness, tight muscles, stomachaches, or even vomiting. GAD can result in missed school days and avoidance of social activities.

Panic disorder is characterized by panic attacks, or episodes of intense fear that occur for no apparent reason. With a panic attack a person may have a sense that things are unreal, and may have physical symptoms like a pounding heart, shortness of breath, dizziness, numbness, or tingling feelings. Sometimes a person having a panic attack mistakenly feels he may be dying or having a heart attack. The panic symptoms are caused by over activity of the body's normal fear response.

Agoraphobia is an intense fear of having a panic attack. People with agoraphobia have had a panic attack before, and worry so much about having another that they avoid going anywhere they think it could possibly occur. They are often left with very few places they feel comfortable going outside their own home.

Social anxiety disorder is an intense fear of social situations. Teens with social anxiety may feel too nervous to raise their hand or talk in class. They may fear making a mistake, saying the wrong answer, or looking foolish. They may feel extremely shy and anxious in situations where they have to interact with others, such as parties, the lunch table, or when they meet new people. They may be overly self-conscious about their clothes or hair, worrying that they might be criticized or teased, or that they might stand out or be noticed. With an extreme form of social anxiety called selective mutism, some kids and teens may be too anxious to talk at all in certain situations.

Obsessive-compulsive disorder (OCD) is characterized by obsessions— thoughts or impulses that occur again and again and that a person feels he can't control—and compulsions—behaviors or rituals that a person feels he must perform to control disturbing thoughts and relieve the anxiety the thoughts trigger. With OCD a teen may, for example, have constant worry and fear about illness or germs, and may become stuck in a pattern of washing and cleaning that becomes time-consuming, distressing, and feels impossible to control. The worries (obsessions) with OCD are unrealistic, but are frightening to the person who has them. For example, a teen with illness obsessions may worry that just by reading about an illness or driving past a hospital he could become ill.

Posttraumatic stress disorder (PTSD) refers to anxiety relating to a traumatic or terrifying past experience. With PTSD, a frightening, life-threatening event such as an accident, serious violence (such as rape, abuse, shooting, or

gang violence), or a natural disas-
ter (such as an earthquake, tornado,
hurricane) causes such a severe fear
response that the person may experience flashbacks, nightmares, or
constant fear, worry, and stress after the fact. PTSD may occur
within days or weeks after the life-
threatening event, or it may be delayed and occur much later.

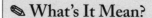

What's It Mean?

Compulsion: Behaviors or rituals that
a person feels he must perform to
control disturbing thoughts and relieve the anxiety the thoughts trigger.

Obsession: Thoughts or impulses
that occur again and again and that
a person feels he can't control.

Phobias are intense unrealistic fears relating to specific situations or things
(that are not actually dangerous), such as heights, dogs, or flying in an airplane. Phobias usually cause people to avoid what they are afraid of. Some
people can work around a phobia if it involves something they do not have
to encounter in their everyday life. Other phobias may involve more common situations or things, and may be harder to steer clear of even if people
do their best to avoid them. Avoiding these things or situations tends to
make the fear stronger each time the person encounters them.

If you have an anxiety disorder, you may feel that it's ruling your life. In
addition to worrying much of the time, you may be easily distracted and
have trouble concentrating. You may feel stressed and tense or unable to
relax. You may experience physical symptoms such as headaches, sweaty hands,
upset stomach, pounding heart, and muscle tension. Like Morgan, you may
find it nearly impossible to fall asleep. Some people have extremely intense
symptoms—for example, people who are experiencing panic attacks may fear
that they are having a heart attack or might even die.

But whether you think you might have an anxiety disorder or you know
someone who does, understanding the disorder and its treatment can help.

Why Do People Get Anxiety Disorders?

There is no one cause for anxiety disorders. Several factors can play a role,
including genetics, brain biochemistry, an overactive "fight or flight" response,
life circumstances, and learned behavior.

Genetics influence a person's brain biochemistry, and may make certain people more prone to problems with anxiety. The brain's biochemistry involves the brain's millions of nerve cells (called neurons) that constantly communicate with each other through chemicals called neurotransmitters.

Neurotransmitters are the brain's chemical messengers, and specific neurotransmitters help to regulate mood. Neurotransmitters are released from one neuron and attach to a receptor on another neuron. Sometimes there is interference with this process, such as if the receptor is blocked and unable to receive the neurotransmitter.

This interference can create an imbalance in the levels of the neurotransmitter in the brain, and can cause symptoms of anxiety. There are many kinds of neurotransmitters; two that are involved in anxiety are called serotonin and dopamine. When there's an imbalance of these chemicals, anxiety and other problems can occur.

Certain things that happen in a person's life can also set the stage for anxiety disorders. Frightening traumatic events that can lead to PTSD are a good example.

Early learning also plays a role. Growing up in a family where others are fearful or anxious can "teach" a child to view the world as a scary place. Likewise, if a child grows up in an environment that is actually scary or dangerous (if there is violence in the child's family or community, for example), the child may learn to be fearful or expect the worst.

♣ It's A Fact!!

Anxiety disorders tend to run in families, suggesting that there is a hereditary, or genetic, component to many of these conditions. A person who has a family member with an anxiety disorder has a greater chance of developing an anxiety disorder, though not necessarily the same type.

The brain's automatic reaction to an anxiety-provoking situation also can fuel an anxiety disorder. Here's how this can happen: when a person senses danger (even if it doesn't turn out to be true danger), the brain quickly reacts by sending a signal to a small structure in the brain called the amygdala (pronounced: uh-mig-duh-luh). The amygdala immediately activates the body's automatic "fight or flight" response, and the body prepares itself for danger. This response is what triggers symptoms like sweating and a pounding heart.

Sometimes it turns out that as soon as the person processes the information in the thinking part of the brain (the cerebral cortex), which happens just moments later, the person realizes there's really no danger. The person then relaxes, and this fight or flight response stops.

But the amygdala is programmed to "remember" the trigger that set this process in motion in case it happens again. This is the brain's attempt to protect the person from future danger by keeping track of all cues that might signal danger. So, for example, if the person encounters the same thing that scared him once before (even if the person later realized it wasn't dangerous), the amygdala may activate the same anxiety reaction. It's possible for the amygdala to begin to overreact, and for the person to mistakenly interpret certain things as dangerous.

How Are Anxiety Disorders Diagnosed And Treated?

Some people go to their medical doctor because they're worried about the physical symptoms associated with anxiety. This is a good idea because symptoms like palpitations, chest pain, stomachaches, vomiting, shortness of breath, shakiness, numbness or tingling, or sleeping problems can be caused by certain medical illnesses.

A doctor can examine a person to determine whether he has any medical conditions that need treatment. But if the doctor doesn't find a medical cause for the symptoms, and sees that there's a certain pattern of physical symptoms, the doctor may diagnose anxiety and refer the person to a mental health specialist.

If you think you may have an anxiety disorder, you need to see a mental health specialist, such as a psychologist or psychiatrist, for an evaluation. Don't wait to ask for help—anxiety can be overwhelming, and it can prevent you from enjoying yourself, your friends, school, and social activities. There are treatments that can help teens with anxiety disorders feel much better, often fairly quickly.

Some people with anxiety try to medicate or relax themselves by using alcohol and drugs (even things like sleeping pills), which may seem to make the anxiety or stress go away temporarily. This is not a good solution for several reasons. Drugs and alcohol create only a false sense of relaxation, can be dangerous, and can lead to lots of other problems, which can make it that much harder to function.

You can expect the mental health specialist to ask about your medical history, your family situation, the symptoms you've been experiencing, and your general well-being. Don't be surprised if some of the questions are very personal—your responses will help the doctor to understand you more fully and create a treatment plan that's right for you.

Treatment for anxiety may include medication, cognitive-behavioral therapy or other types of talk therapy, and relaxation or biofeedback to control tense muscles. A combination of treatments may be prescribed.

When medications are part of the treatment for anxiety, often a certain class of medications called SSRIs [selective serotonin reuptake inhibitors] is used. This is sometimes confusing to people with anxiety because the SSRI medications are commonly referred to as "antidepressants."

Here's the scoop to clear up the confusion: the SSRI medications were first developed as antidepressants, but it was recognized that they also have anti-anxiety effects. So, how could they work for both? Because depression and anxiety both involve, among other things, an imbalance of the neurotransmitter serotonin. SSRI medications help to restore the normal balance of serotonin, and therefore help with both depression and anxiety.

Though not every teen who has an anxiety disorder needs medication (in fact, most don't), the right medication can help to reduce symptoms of anxiety, and can be a great relief to someone whose anxiety symptoms are causing tremendous distress. Often when doctors prescribe medication, they begin with a very small dosage, and gradually increase to the dosage that works best. It may take some time to get the dosage that works best for you. And it may take several weeks before the full benefits of a certain medication are felt. As with any medication, it's very important to take it exactly as prescribed and to tell your doctor about any side effects.

In psychotherapy, or talk therapy, a teen talks with a mental health professional about the stresses and anxiety he's feeling. Getting support and sorting through problems by talking them through can be helpful to teens with anxiety.

In a particular type of talk therapy called cognitive-behavioral therapy (CBT), teens take an active role in "unlearning" some of their fear. CBT helps teens learn new ways to think and act when confronted with anxiety, and to manage and deal with stress so it doesn't get out of hand. In CBT, teens learn how to detect and measure their anxiety, recognize what triggers it, and practice ways to reduce it. They learn what makes their fear worse and what can ease it. Techniques vary, but may include relaxation and breathing exercises or exposure therapy, where a person is gradually exposed what triggers his fear. If it's done with proper support and new coping skills, exposure helps even intense fear fade away.

Dealing With An Anxiety Disorder

If you have an anxiety disorder, it may be difficult for your friends or family to understand just how you feel. Sometimes people give unrealistic advice—like telling you to just stop worrying. Though they may have the best intentions, they may not understand that it's not that simple. You may have to explain this to them.

Because others may not always understand, sometimes people are reluctant to let loved ones know what they are going through. Some people may be concerned that their fear or behavior may be seen as childish, silly, or weird. But communication is the key. Close friends and family can be part of the solution, and their care and support can be valuable. Let them know what they can do to help.

If you know someone who has an anxiety disorder, be a supportive friend. If your friend goes to a support group, you might offer to go to one of the meetings too. Tell your friend you're there to listen if he or she would like to talk.

✔ Quick Tip
Don't hesitate to tell your doctor or therapist about what's working and what isn't—you're a member of your treatment team, and your ideas and feelings are important.

Chapter 13

Post-Traumatic Stress Disorder Can Lead To Sleep Disturbances

Many people suffer from problems with their sleep. This can be especially true for those who have witnessed or experienced one or more traumatic events such as rape, military combat, natural disasters, beatings, or neighborhood violence. Some individuals exposed to traumatic physical or psychological events develop a condition known as post-traumatic stress disorder (PTSD). It is well known that a problem with sleep is one of many problems for those with PTSD. Sleep problems, such as difficulty falling asleep, waking frequently, and having distressing dreams or nightmares, are common to those with PTSD. In fact, sleep disturbance can be a normal response to past trauma or anticipated threat.

What are the major reasons why people with PTSD have problems with sleep?

Severe psychological or physical trauma can cause changes in a person's basic biological functioning. As a result of being traumatized, a person with PTSD may be constantly hyper-vigilant, or "on the lookout," to protect him- or herself from danger. It is difficult to have restful sleep when you feel the need to be always alert.

About This Chapter: "Sleep and Posttraumatic Stress Disorder (PTSD)," National Center for Posttraumatic Stress disorder, U.S. Department of Veterans Affairs (www.ncptsd.va.gov), April 6, 2007.

What are some sleep problems commonly associated with PTSD?

Difficulty Falling Asleep

- *Basic Biological Changes:* Actual biological changes may occur as a result of trauma, making it difficult to fall asleep. In addition, a continued state of hyper-arousal or watchfulness is usually present. It is very hard for people to fall asleep if they think and feel that they need to stay awake and alert to protect themselves (and possibly others) from danger.

- *Medical Problems:* There are medical conditions commonly associated with PTSD. They can make going to sleep difficult. Such problems include: chronic pain, stomach and intestinal problems, and pelvic-area problems (in women).

- *Your Thoughts:* A person's thoughts can also contribute to problems with sleep. For example, thinking about the traumatic event, thinking about general worries and problems, or just thinking, "Here we go again, another night, another terrible night's sleep," may make it difficult to fall asleep.

- *Use Of Drugs Or Alcohol:* These substances are often associated with difficulty going to sleep.

Difficulty Staying Asleep

- *Distressing Dreams Or Nightmares:* Nightmares are typical for people with PTSD. Usually, the nightmares tend to be about the traumatic event or some aspect of it. For example, in Vietnam veterans, nightmares are usually about traumatic things that happened in combat. In dreams, the person with PTSD may also attempt to express the dominant emotions of the traumatic event; these are usually fear and terror. For example, it is not uncommon to dream about being overwhelmed by a tidal wave or swept up by a whirlwind.

- *Thrashing Movements:* Because of overall hyper-arousal, active movements of the arms or legs during bad dreams or nightmares may cause awakening. For example, if one were having a dream about fleeing an aggressor, one might wake up because of the physical movements of trying to run away.

- *Anxiety (Panic) Attacks:* Attacks of anxiety or outright panic may interrupt sleep. Symptoms of such attacks may include:
  - Feeling your heart beating very fast
  - Feeling that your heart is "skipping a beat"
  - Feeling lightheaded or dizzy
  - Having difficulty breathing (tight chest, pressure on chest)
  - Sweating
  - Feeling really hot ("hot flashes")
  - Feeling really cold (cold sweat)
  - Feeling fearful
  - Feeling disoriented or confused
  - Fearing that you may die (as a result of these symptoms)
  - Thinking and feeling that you may be "going crazy"
  - Thinking and feeling that you may "lose control"

- *Hearing The Slightest Sound And Waking Up To Check For Safety:* Many people with PTSD, especially combat veterans, wake up frequently during the night. This can be for various reasons. However, once awake, a "perimeter check," or a check of the area, is often made. For example, a Vet may get up, check the sleeping area, check the locks on windows and doors, and even go outside and walk around to check for danger. Then the Vet may stay awake and vigilant and "stand guard;" he (or she) may not return to sleep that night.

What can you do if you have problems sleeping due to PTSD?

Talk To Your Doctor

- Let your doctor know that you have trouble sleeping. Tell your doctor exactly what the problems are; he or she can help you best if you share this information about yourself.

- Let your doctor know that you have (or think you have) PTSD. It is not your fault that you have these symptoms. Tell your doctor exactly what they are.

- Let your doctor know about any physical problems that you think are contributing to your sleep problems. For example, chronic pain associated with traumatic injuries can make it difficult to sleep.

> ### ✎ What's It Mean?
>
> Night Terrors: These are events such as screaming or shaking while asleep. The person may appear awake to an observer, but he or she is not responsive. Night terrors are commonly associated with post-traumatic stress disorder (PTSD).

- Let your doctor know about any other emotional problems you have—these may also be contributing to your sleep problems. For example, depression or panic attacks can make it hard to fall asleep or to stay asleep.

Your doctor may recommend that you work with a therapist skilled in dealing with emotional and behavioral problems. Psychologists, social workers, and psychiatrists fall into this category. They can help you take a closer look at, and possibly change, the variety of factors that may be preventing you from sleeping well. They can help you with PTSD and other problems.

Do Not Use Alcohol Or Other Drugs

These substances disturb a variety of bodily processes. They impair a person's ability to get a good night's sleep. For example, alcohol may help a person fall asleep, but it interferes with one's ability to stay asleep.

If you are dependent on drugs or alcohol, let your doctor know, and seek assistance for this problem.

Other Strategies

- Limit substances that contain caffeine (soda, coffee, some over-the-counter medicines).

- Try to set a regular sleep/wake schedule: A consistent sleep schedule helps to regulate and set the body's "internal clock," which tells us when we are tired and when it is time to sleep, among other things.

- Make your sleeping area as free from distractions as possible: Aim for quiet surroundings; keep the room darkened; keep the television out of the bedroom.

- Consider a light nighttime snack: A light snack after dinner may prevent hunger from waking you up in the middle of the night.

- Avoid over-arousal for at least 2–3 hours prior to going to sleep: Try not to get your body and mind in "arousal mode." Things that may tend to do this are: heavy meals, strenuous exercise, heated arguments, paying bills, and action-packed movies.

- Don't worry that you can't sleep: Remember, there may be a number of reasons for your sleep problems. The first step is to talk to your doctor.

♣ It's A Fact!!

There are a number of medications that are helpful for sleep problems in PTSD. Depending on your sleep symptoms and other factors, your doctor may prescribe some medication for you.

Chapter 14

Sleeping Pills: Benefits And Risks

People with insomnia often turn first to sleeping pills for a quick fix to help them fall asleep and stay asleep. Sleep medications may seem to help the problem at first, but they do not cure insomnia and often lose effectiveness over the long term. In addition, sleeping pills have side-effects and can be addictive.

Sleeping pills (or sleep medications) fall into two categories:

• Over-the-counter (OTC) sleep medications

• Prescription sleeping pills

What are the benefits and risks of over-the-counter sleep medications?

You can walk into a drugstore and choose from an array of sleep aids, offered without prescription. The main ingredient of over-the-counter sleeping pills is an antihistamine. Antihistamines are generally taken for allergies, but they also make you feel very sleepy. Common over-the-counter sleep medications are Sleep-Eze, Sominex, Nytol, and Unison; they contain antihistamines such as:

- diphenhydramine hydrochloride,

- diphenhydramine citrate, or

- doxylamine succinate.

In general, over-the-counter sleep medications are not a good choice because they:

- Are not intended for long-term use.

> **♣ It's A Fact!!**
>
> Extended use of sleep medications often makes insomnia worse over the long term. Prescription sleep medications can be habit-forming and often do not treat the specific cause of the insomnia.
>
> Source: © 2007 Helpguide.org.

- Interfere with mental alertness during the day, so you should avoid driving and other similar tasks. You may also be at risk for falling.

- Reduce the quality of your sleep by reducing time you spend in deep sleep.

Use over-the-counter sleep medications only for transient or short-term insomnia and in conjunction with changes to your sleeping habits. Be sure to pay attention to your body's physical response to these sleep medications. Immediately discontinue use if you experience any severe adverse effects.

Common side effects of over-the-counter sleeping pills:

- drowsiness the next day

- dizziness

- lack of coordination

- forgetfulness

- constipation

- urinary retention

- blurred vision, and

- dry mouth and throat

In addition, you can develop a tolerance for over-the-counter sleep aids after using them for just a few days. You may find quickly that you need a higher dosage to accomplish the same effect. As with any medication, it is advisable to consult with your doctor before taking over-the-counter sleep medications.

Why are sleep medications often prescribed for the treatment of insomnia?

Many people experiencing sleep problems want a quick fix for their problems. But the causes of insomnia are complex and vary by person. Several of the successful behavioral treatments for insomnia are time-intensive and require a lot of work by the person experiencing insomnia. The thought of a pill that can solve the problem quickly is very appealing. Unfortunately, sleep medications don't cure insomnia, and they can often exacerbate the problem over the long term.

If you want to take medications to help you sleep because you are in a great deal of pain, are traveling, or just need to get some sleep, pay attention to the type of medication you choose and try to use the medication only when you really need it. If you also commit to making your sleep habits and sleep environment more conducive to sleep, you can limit the effects of insomnia on your life.

What are the dangers of sleep medications for treating insomnia?

Because sleep medications do not address the root cause of insomnia, they can become a crutch to lean on, rather than a cure. Just as you would not leave a cast on a broken bone indefinitely because it would cause the muscle to atrophy, sleep medications should be seen as a temporary aid for sleep problems, not a long-term solution.

Other concerns about the use of both over-the-counter and prescription sleep medications include the following:

- development of drug tolerance
- development of drug dependence
- physical side effects
- interactions with other drugs or chemicals in the body
- withdrawal symptoms
- rebound insomnia

What are the types of prescription sleep medications?

The following is a list of commonly prescribed sleep medications:

Short-Acting Sedative-Hypnotics (Non-Benzodiazepines)

This class of medications causes you to feel sleepy by increasing the normal effects of the brain chemical gamma-aminobutyric acid (GABA). They are more effective and safer for long-term, nightly use than benzodiazepines. However, they may lead to addiction. Some popular medications in this class are:

- zolpidem (Ambien)

- zaleplon (Sonata)

- eszopiclone (Lunesta)

Melatonin Receptor Agonists

This newer hypnotic reduces alertness by acting on the melatonin receptors in the brain. It's used for sleep onset problems. The medication has some side-effects, but is not a narcotic. It is not effective for problems in staying asleep.

- ramelteon (Rozerem)

Benzodiazepines (Tranquilizers)

This class of medications works by slowing down the central nervous system to cause drowsiness. They are effective only for a few weeks and may lead to drug-dependence, impairment in memory and movement, and a hangover the next day. These drugs are now less frequently prescribed than non-benzodiazepines. Some popular medications in this class are:

- flurazepam (Dalmane)

- temazepam (Restoril)

- estazolam (ProSom)

Other Sleep Medications: In addition, sedating antidepressants are sometimes prescribed for insomnia. These medications are primarily for the treatment of depression, but have sedating side-effects. Sedating antidepressants have more negative effects than the sedative-hypnotics and are generally best prescribed only for insomnia in the context of depression. Note that all antidepressants carry the risk of serious side-effects. An example is trazodone (Desyrel).

Older sleep medications are the barbiturates, no longer recommended for insomnia treatment. Barbiturates include Phenobarbital and come with a high risk of overdose, addiction, and abuse.

How long should drug treatment last?

Sleep medications are meant to provide temporary relief from insomnia, not a long-term solution. The safety of long-term use of sleeping pills has not been established. Changes in your sleep habits and sleep environment, plus behavioral therapies, provide a better long-term solution to insomnia.

If you take sleep medications, the National Sleep Foundation recommends that you:

- begin with the lowest possible effective dose;
- use the drugs on a short-term basis, if you use them nightly;
- take the drugs intermittently, if you use them long-term; and
- use the drugs only in combination with good sleep hygiene and/or behavioral treatments.

✔ Quick Tip

If you decide to try prescription sleep medications, it is wise to discuss the decision with your doctor and:

- Educate yourself thoroughly about the drugs available, the potential side effects, and any interactions with other medications you take.

- Follow directions closely, starting with a very small dose and increasing gradually, according to the doctor's schedule.

- Pay attention to your body, emotions, and actions to determine if any negative side effects are occurring.

- Use the medications intermittently, rather than nightly, in order to decrease the negative effects and to increase the effectiveness when you do use them.

- Ask your doctor for specific instructions for decreasing and/or terminating use.

Source: © 2007 Helpguide.org.

Chapter 15

Cognitive Behavior Therapy For Treating Sleep Problems

Findings

More sleep would make most people happier, healthier and safer. But for people with sleep disorders, trying to get more sleep can be a nightmarish experience. Surveys conducted by the National Sleep Foundation reveal that at least 40 million Americans suffer from over 70 different sleep disorders and 60 percent of adults report having sleep problems a few nights a week or more. Sleep disorders and sleep disturbances comprise a broad range of problems, including sleep apnea, narcolepsy, insomnia, jet-lag syndrome, and disturbed biological and circadian rhythms.

For the estimated one in 10 people who suffer from chronic insomnia, psychologists are helping them get a good night's sleep through the benefits of cognitive behavioral therapy (CBT). In a 2001 study published in the *Journal of the American Medical Association* (*JAMA*), psychologist Jack Edinger, PhD, and colleagues found the CBT worked better than either progressive muscle relaxation or a placebo treatment for people with insomnia. Another *JAMA* study two years earlier by psychologist Charles Morin, PhD, found that behavioral and pharmacological therapies, alone or in combination, are effective in the short-term management of late life insomnia. But those who received CBT had the best long-term results and the participants rated the behavioral therapy as more effective and satisfying. A 2001 German study by Jutta Backhaus and colleagues found that the benefits of short-term CBT had long-term effects. After therapy the participants improved their total sleep time and sleep efficiency and reduced their sleep latency and negative sleep-related cognitions, and those improvements were sustained during the three-year follow-up period.

How does cognitive behavioral therapy help people sleep better? Research shows that CBT reduces false beliefs about sleep (the cognitive part) and also addresses the behavioral aspect, such as what to do when you are lying in bed and can't fall asleep. A 2002 study by Dr. Morin highlighting people's misconceptions about sleep found those that who received CBT reduced their false beliefs, which resulted in increases in the amount of time they spend in bed actually sleeping. Misconceptions regarding sleep can involve unrealistic expectations about sleep ("I must get 8 hours of sleep every night"), exaggeration of the consequences of not getting enough sleep ("If I don't get a full 8 hours of sleep tonight a catastrophe will happen"), faulty thinking about the cause of your insomnia ("My insomnia is completely caused by a biochemical imbalance"), and misconceptions about health sleep practices.

> **♣ It's A Fact!!**
> Cognitive behavioral therapy is becoming the "treatment of choice" for many people with insomnia.

A 2004 study by psychologist Célyne Bastien, PhD, and colleagues found that group therapy and telephone consultations using cognitive-behavioral therapy was a cost-effective alternative to individual therapy for the management of insomnia. All three CBT treatment methods produced improvements in sleep that were maintained for six months after the treatment period ended.

Significance

Up to 40 percent of adults report at least occasional difficulty sleeping, and the National Institutes of Health reports that chronic and severe forms of insomnia affects between 10 to 15 percents of adults. Even small disruptions in sleep can wreak havoc on human safety and performance. Estimates by the National Highway Traffic Safety Administration indicate that drowsy or fatigued driving leads to more than 100,000 motor vehicle crashes per year.

Practical Application

Findings from controlled clinical trials indicate that 70 to 80 percent of insomnia patients benefit from cognitive-behavioral interventions. Although CBT is now considered the treatment of choice for chronic insomnia, no single treatment method is effective for all insomnia patients, so behavioral and pharmacological approaches sometimes need to be integrated.

More and more sleep disorder clinics are popping up across the country—there are now more than 300, with most hospitals offering sleep clinics. Look for those that offer more than just pharmacological treatment options.

Here are some tips for anyone, including those without serious sleep problems, that is looking for ways to get a good night's sleep:

- Restrict the amount of time spent in bed as close as possible to the actual sleep time

- Go to bed only when sleepy, not just fatigue but sleepy

- If unable to sleep (for example, within 20 min), get out of bed and go to another room and return to bed only when sleep is imminent

- Use the bed and bedroom for sleep (and sex) only; no eating, TV watching, radio listening, planning, or problem solving in bed

- Maintain a regular sleep schedule, particularly a strict arising time every morning regardless of the amount of sleep the night before

- Avoid daytime napping

Cited Research

Backhaus, J., Hohagen, F., Voderholzer, U., Riemann, D. (2001). Long-term effectiveness of a short-term cognitive-behavioral group treatment for primary insomnia. *European Archives of Psychiatry & Clinical Neuroscience*, Vol. 251, No. 1, pp. 35–41.

Bastien, C.H., Morin, C.M., Ouellet, M., Blais, F.C., Bouchard, S. (2004). Cognitive-behavioral therapy for insomnia: Comparison of individual therapy, group therapy, and telephone consultations. *Journal of Consulting and Clinical Psychology*, Vol. 72, No. 4, pp. 63–659.

Edinger, J.D., Wohlgemuth, W.K., Radtke, R.A., Marsh, G.R., Quillian, R.E. (2001). Cognitive behavioral therapy for treatment of chronic primary insomnia: A randomized controlled trial. *Journal of the American Medical Association*, Vol. 285, No. 14, pp. 1856–1864.

Morin, C.M. (2002). Contributions of cognitive-behavioral approaches to the clinical management of insomnia. *Primary Care Companion, Journal of Clinical Psychiatry* (suppl 1), pp. 21–26.

Morin, C.M., Blais, F., Savard, J. (2002). Are changes in beliefs and attitudes about sleep related to sleep improvements in the treatment of insomnia? *Behaviour Research & Therapy*, Vol. 40, No. 7, pp. 741–752.

Morin, C.M., Colecchi, C., Stone, J., Sood, R., Brink, D. (1999). Behavioral and pharmacological therapies for late-life insomnia: A randomized controlled trial. *Journal of the American Medical Association*, Vol. 281, No. 11, pp. 991–999.

Chapter 16

Complementary And Alternative Therapies For Sleep Problems

A recent analysis of national survey data reveals that over 1.6 million American adults use some form of complementary and alternative medicine (CAM) to treat insomnia or trouble sleeping[1] according to scientists at the National Center for Complementary and Alternative Medicine (NCCAM), part of the National Institutes of Health. The data came from the 2002 National Health Interview Survey (NHIS) conducted by the National Center for Health Statistics of the Centers for Disease Control and Prevention.

In 2002 the NHIS, an in-person, annual health survey, included over 31,000 U.S. adults aged 18 years and older. A CAM supplement to the survey asked about the use of 27 types of CAM therapies, as well as a variety of medical conditions for which CAM may be used, including insomnia or trouble sleeping. Survey results show that over 17 percent of adults reported trouble sleeping or insomnia in the past 12 months. Of those with insomnia or trouble sleeping, 4.5 percent—more than 1.6 million people—used some form of CAM to treat their condition.

About This Chapter: This chapter begins with "Over 1.6 Million Americans Use CAM for Insomnia or Trouble Sleeping," National Center for Complementary and Alternative Medicine (nccam.nih.gov), October 10, 2006. It continues with "AHRQ Issues New Report on the Safety and Effectiveness of Melatonin Supplements," Agency for Healthcare Research and Quality (www.ahrq.gov), December 8, 2004. It concludes with "Questions and Answers About Valerian for Insomnia and Other Sleep Disorders," Office of Dietary Supplements (ods.od.nih.gov), April 13, 2006.

"These data offer some new insights regarding the prevalence of insomnia or trouble sleeping in the United States and the types of CAM therapies people use to treat these conditions," said Dr. Margaret A. Chesney, Acting Director of NCCAM. "They will help us develop new research questions regarding the safety and efficacy of the CAM therapies being used."

Those using CAM to treat insomnia or trouble sleeping were more likely to use biologically based therapies (nearly 65 percent), such as herbal therapies, or mind-body therapies (more than 39 percent), such as relaxation techniques. A majority of people who used herbal or relaxation therapies for their insomnia reported that they were helpful. The two most common reasons people gave for using CAM to treat insomnia were they thought it would be interesting to try (nearly 67 percent) and they thought CAM combined with a conventional treatment would be helpful (nearly 64 percent).

♣ **It's A Fact!!**
Additional Facts From The National Health Interview Survey

- Nearly 61 percent of those reporting trouble sleeping were women versus about 39 percent men.

- Insomnia peaks in middle age (45–64 years old), and a second increase appears in people 85 and older.

- African Americans and Asians appear less likely to report trouble sleeping or insomnia than whites.

- Those with higher education also are less likely to report insomnia or trouble sleeping.

Source: National Center for Complementary and Alternative Medicine, 2006.

In addition to looking at the data on CAM use and insomnia, the researchers also looked at the connection between trouble sleeping and five significant health conditions: diabetes, hypertension, congestive heart failure, anxiety and depression, and obesity. They found that insomnia or trouble sleeping is highly associated with four of the five conditions: hypertension, congestive heart failure, anxiety and depression, and obesity.

Reference

1. Pearson NJ, Johnson LL, Nahin RL. Insomnia, Trouble Sleeping, and Complementary and Alternative Medicine: Analysis of the 2002 National Health Interview Survey Data. *Archives of Internal Medicine*, 2006; 166:1775–1782.

AHRQ Issues New Report On The Safety And Effectiveness Of Melatonin Supplements

A new evidence review by HHS' (Health and Human Services) Agency for Healthcare Research and Quality (AHRQ) found that melatonin supplements, which people often take for problems sleeping, appear to be safe when used over a period of days or weeks, at relatively high doses and in various formulations. However, the safety of melatonin supplements used over months or even years is unclear. While there is some evidence for benefits of melatonin supplements, for most sleep disorders the authors found evidence suggesting limited or no benefits. But the authors say that firm conclusions cannot be drawn until more research is conducted. The report was requested and funded by the National Center for Complementary and Alternative Medicine, a part of HHS' National Institutes of Health.

The report's authors reviewed the scientific evidence to date for the benefits of melatonin supplements used for disorders due to sleep schedule alterations and primary and secondary sleep disorders. Disorders due to sleep schedule alterations can stem from flying across time zones or working night shifts. Primary sleep disorders, which include insomnia, can be caused by factors such as stress or drinking too much caffeinated coffee. Secondary sleep disorders can also include insomnia, but patients in this category also have underlying mental disorders, such as psychoses or mood and anxiety disorders, neurological conditions such as dementia and Parkinson disease, or chronic pulmonary disease.

Among those problems for which melatonin supplements appear to provide little benefit are jet lag—a problem that often nags coast-to-coast travelers and those who fly through other time zones, as well as people who work night shifts.

In contrast, the authors found evidence to suggest that melatonin supplements may be effective when used in the short term to treat delayed sleep phase syndrome in persons with primary sleep disorders. In delayed sleep phase syndrome, a person's internal biological clock becomes "out of sync," making it difficult to fall asleep until very late at night and to wake up early the next morning. But melatonin supplements may decrease sleep onset latency—the time it takes to fall asleep after going to bed—in persons with primary sleep disorders such as insomnia, although the magnitude of the effect appears to be limited.

> ♣ **It's A Fact!!**
>
> In its natural form, melatonin is produced by the brain's pineal gland to regulate the sleep cycle. In the evening the level of the hormone in the bloodstream rises sharply, reducing alertness and inviting sleep, and in the morning it falls back, encouraging waking.
>
> Source: Agency for Healthcare Research and Quality, 2004.

Melatonin supplements do not appear to have an effect on sleep efficiency in persons with primary sleep disorders, and the effects of the hormone do not seem to vary by the individual's age, type of primary sleep disorder, dose, or length of treatment. Sleep efficiency refers to the percent of time a person is asleep after going to bed. Furthermore, melatonin supplements do not appear to affect sleep quality, wakefulness after sleep onset, total sleep time or percent of time spent in rapid eye movement (REM) sleep.

In people with secondary sleep disorders, melatonin supplements do not appear to have an impact on sleep latency in either adults or children—regardless of dose or duration of treatment. On the other hand, the hormone

---

✎ What's It Mean?

REM sleep: This most important phase of sleep is characterized by extensive physiological changes such as accelerated breathing, increased brain activity, REM (rapid eye movement), and muscle relaxation.

Source: Agency for Healthcare Research and Quality, 2004.

does appear to increase sleep efficiency modestly, but not enough to be considered clinically significant. Melatonin supplements were not found to have an effect on wakefulness after sleep onset or percent of time spent in REM sleep, but they do appear to increase total sleep time.

Questions And Answers About Valerian For Insomnia And Other Sleep Disorders

What is valerian?

Valerian (*Valeriana officinalis*), a member of the Valerianaceae family, is a perennial plant native to Europe and Asia and naturalized in North America. It has a distinctive odor that many find unpleasant. Other names include setwall (English), *Valerianae radix* (Latin), Baldrianwurzel (German), and phu (Greek). The genus *Valerian* includes over 250 species, but *V. officinalis* is the species most often used in the United States and Europe and is the only species discussed in this fact sheet.

What are common valerian preparations?

Preparations of valerian marketed as dietary supplements are made from its roots, rhizomes (underground stems), and stolons (horizontal stems). Dried roots are prepared as teas or tinctures, and dried plant materials and extracts are put into capsules or incorporated into tablets.

There is no scientific agreement as to the active constituents of valerian, and its activity may result from interactions among multiple constituents rather than any one compound or class of compounds. The content of volatile oils, including valerenic acids; the less volatile sesquiterpenes; or the valepotriates (esters of short-chain fatty acids) is sometimes used to standardize valerian extracts. As with most herbal preparations, many other compounds are also present.

What are the historical uses of valerian?

Valerian has been used as a medicinal herb since at least the time of ancient Greece and Rome. Its therapeutic uses were described by Hippocrates, and in the 2nd century, Galen prescribed valerian for insomnia. In the 16th century, it was used to treat nervousness, trembling, headaches, and heart palpitations. In the mid-19th century, valerian was considered a stimulant that caused some of the same complaints it is thought to treat and was generally held in low esteem as a medicinal herb. During World War II, it was used in England to relieve the stress of air raids.

In addition to sleep disorders, valerian has been used for gastrointestinal spasms and distress, epileptic seizures, and attention deficit hyperactivity disorder. However, scientific evidence is not sufficient to support the use of valerian for these conditions.

Have clinical studies been done on valerian and sleep disorders?

Although the results of some studies suggest that valerian may be useful for insomnia and other sleep disorders, results of other studies do not. Interpretation of these studies is complicated by the fact the studies had small sample sizes, used different amounts and sources of valerian, measured different outcomes, or did not consider potential bias resulting from high participant withdrawal rates. Overall, the evidence from these trials for the sleep-promoting effects of valerian is inconclusive.

What is the regulatory status of valerian in the United States?

In the United States, valerian is sold as a dietary supplement, and dietary supplements are regulated as foods, not drugs. Therefore, pre-market evaluation and approval by the Food and Drug Administration are not required unless claims are made for specific disease prevention or treatment. Because dietary supplements are not always tested for manufacturing consistency, the composition may vary considerably between manufacturing lots.

Can valerian be harmful?

Few adverse events attributable to valerian have been reported for clinical study participants. Headaches, dizziness, pruritus, and gastrointestinal disturbances are the most common effects reported in clinical trials but similar effects were also reported for the placebo. In one study an increase in sleepiness was noted the morning after 900 mg of valerian was taken. Investigators from another study concluded that 600 mg of valerian (LI 156) did not have a clinically significant effect on reaction time, alertness, and concentration the morning after ingestion. Several case reports described adverse effects, but in one case where suicide was attempted with a massive overdose it is not possible to clearly attribute the symptoms to valerian.

Valepotriates, which are a component of valerian but are not necessarily present in commercial preparations, had cytotoxic activity in vitro but were not carcinogenic in animal studies.

Who should not take valerian?

• Women who are pregnant or nursing should not take valerian without medical advice because the possible risks to the fetus or infant have not been evaluated.

• Children younger than 3 years old should not take valerian because the possible risks to children of this age have not been evaluated.

• Individuals taking valerian should be aware of the theoretical possibility of additive sedative effects from alcohol or sedative drugs, such as barbiturates and benzodiazepines.

Does valerian interact with any drugs or affect laboratory tests?

Although valerian has not been reported to interact with any drugs or to influence laboratory tests, this has not been rigorously studied.

What are some additional sources of scientific information on valerian?

Medical libraries are a source of information about medicinal herbs. Other sources include web-based resources such as PubMed available at http://www.ncbi.nlm.nih.gov/entrez/query.fcgi?holding=nih.

For general information on botanicals and their use as dietary supplements, please see Background Information About Botanical Dietary Supplements (http://ods.od.nih.gov/factsheets/botanicalbackground.asp) and General Background Information About Dietary Supplements (http://ods.od.nih.gov/factsheets/dietarysupplements.asp), from the Office of Dietary Supplements (ODS).

☞ Remember!!

- Valerian is an herb sold as a dietary supplement in the United States.

- Valerian is a common ingredient in products promoted as mild sedatives and sleep aids for nervous tension and insomnia.

- Evidence from clinical studies of the efficacy of valerian in treating sleep disorders such as insomnia is inconclusive.

- Constituents of valerian have been shown to have sedative effects in animals, but there is no scientific agreement on valerian's mechanisms of action.

- Although few adverse events have been reported, long-term safety data are not available.

Source: Office of Dietary Supplements, 2006.

Part Three

Sleep Disorders And Related Problems

Chapter 17

Common Sleep Problems

Garrett had a hard time waking up for school during his sophomore year. At first he thought it was because he'd been going to bed late over summer vacation and then sleeping in the next day. He assumed he'd adjust to his school schedule after a couple of weeks. But as the school year progressed, Garrett found himself lying awake in bed until 2 or 3 in the morning, even though he got up at 6:30 A.M. every day. He began falling asleep in class and his grades started to suffer.

Most teens don't get enough sleep, but that's usually because they're overloaded and tend to skimp on sleep. But sleep problems can keep some teens, like Garrett, awake at night even when they want to sleep.

Over time, those nights of missed sleep (whether they're caused by a sleep disorder or simply not scheduling enough time for the necessary ZZZs) can build into a sleep deficit. People with a sleep deficit are unable to concentrate, study, and work effectively. They can also experience emotional problems, like depression.

What Happens During Sleep?

You don't notice it, of course, but while you're asleep, your brain is still active. As people sleep, their brains pass through five stages of sleep. Together,

About This Chapter: This information was provided by TeensHealth, one of the largest resources online for medically reviewed health information written for parents, kids, and teens. For more articles like this one, visit www.TeensHealth.org, or www.KidsHealth.org. © 2004 The Nemours Foundation.

stages 1, 2, 3, 4, and REM (rapid eye movement) sleep make up a sleep cycle. One complete sleep cycle lasts about 90 to 100 minutes. So during an average night's sleep, a person will experience about four or five cycles of sleep.

Stages 1 and 2 are periods of light sleep from which a person can easily be awakened. During these stages, eye movements slow down and eventually stop, heart and breathing rates slow down, and body temperature decreases. Stages 3 and 4 are deep sleep stages. It's more difficult to awaken someone during these stages, and when awakened, a person will often feel groggy and disoriented for a few minutes. Stages 3 and 4 are the most refreshing of the sleep stages—it is this type of sleep that we crave when we are very tired.

The final stage of the sleep cycle is known as REM sleep because of the rapid eye movements that occur during this stage. During REM sleep, other physical changes take place—breathing becomes rapid, the heart beats faster, and the limb muscles don't move. This is the stage of sleep when a person has the most vivid dreams.

Why Do Teens Have Trouble Sleeping?

Research shows that teens need 8½ to more than 9 hours of sleep a night. You don't need to be a math whiz to figure out that if you wake up for school at 6:00 A.M., you'd have to go to bed at 9:00 P.M. to reach the 9-hour mark. Studies have found that many teens, like Garrett, have trouble falling asleep that early, though. It's not because they don't want to sleep. It's because their brains naturally work on later schedules and aren't ready for bed.

Changes in the body clock aren't the only reason teens lose sleep, though. Lots of

♣ It's A Fact!!

During adolescence, the body's circadian rhythm (sort of like an internal biological clock) is reset, telling a teen to fall asleep later at night and wake up later in the morning. This change in the circadian rhythm seems to be due to the fact that the brain hormone is produced later at night in teens than it is for kids and adults, making it harder for teens to fall asleep. This phenomenon has a medical name: delayed sleep phase syndrome. Although it's common, delayed sleep phase syndrome doesn't affect every teen.

people have insomnia—trouble falling or staying asleep. The most common cause of insomnia is stress. But all sorts of things can lead to insomnia, including physical discomfort (the stuffy nose of a cold or the pain of a headache, for example), emotional troubles (like family problems or relationship difficulties), and even sleeping environment (a room that's too hot, cold, or noisy).

It's common for everyone to have insomnia from time to time. But if insomnia lasts for a month or longer with no relief, then doctors consider it chronic. Chronic insomnia can be caused by problems like depression. People with chronic insomnia can often get help for their condition from a doctor, therapist, or other counselor.

For some people, insomnia can be made worse by worrying about the insomnia itself. A brief period of insomnia can build into something longer lasting when a person becomes anxious about not sleeping or worried about feeling tired the next day. Doctors call this psychophysiologic insomnia.

A number of other conditions can disrupt sleep in teens, including:

Periodic Limb Movement Disorder And Restless Legs Syndrome

People with these conditions find their sleep is disrupted by leg (or, less frequently, arm) movements, leaving them tired or irritable from lack of sleep. In the case of periodic limb movement disorder (PLMD), these movements are involuntary twitches or jerks: They're called involuntary because the person isn't consciously controlling them and is often unaware of the movement. People with restless legs syndrome (RLS) actually feel physical sensations in their limbs, such as tingling, itching, cramping, or burning. The only way they can relieve these feelings is by moving their legs or arms to get rid of the discomfort.

Doctors can treat PLMD and RLS. For some people, treating an iron deficiency makes RLS go away; other people may need to take other types of medication.

Obstructive Sleep Apnea

This sleep disorder causes a person to stop breathing temporarily during sleep. One common cause of obstructive sleep apnea is enlarged tonsils or adenoids (tissues located in the passage that connects the nose and throat).

Being overweight or obese can also lead a person to develop obstructive sleep apnea.

People with obstructive sleep apnea may snore, have difficulty breathing, and even sweat heavily during sleep. Because it disrupts sleep, someone with sleep apnea may feel extremely sleepy or irritable during the day. People who show signs of obstructive sleep apnea, such as loud snoring or excessive daytime sleepiness, should be evaluated by a doctor.

Reflux

Some people have gastro-esophageal reflux disease (GERD), which causes stomach acid to move backward up into the esophagus, producing the uncomfortable, burning sensation known as heartburn. GERD symptoms can be worse when someone is lying down. Even if someone doesn't notice the feelings of heartburn during sleep, the discomfort it causes can still interfere with the sleep cycle.

Nightmares

Most teens have nightmares on occasion, but frequent nightmares can disrupt sleep patterns by waking someone during the

---

✔ **Quick Tip**
What Should I Do?

If you're getting enough rest at night and you're still feeling tired during the day, it's a good idea to visit your doctor. Excessive tiredness can be caused by all sorts of health problems, not just difficulties with sleep.

If your doctor suspects a sleep problem, he or she will look at your overall health and sleep habits. In addition to doing a physical examination, the doctor will take your medical history by asking you about any concerns and symptoms you have, your past health, your family's health, any medications you're taking, any allergies you may have, and other issues. The doctor may also do tests to find out whether any conditions—such as obstructive sleep apnea—might be interfering with your sleep.

Different sleep problems are treated differently. Some can be treated with medications, whereas others can be helped by special techniques such as light therapy (where someone sits in front of a light box for a certain amount of time each day) or other practices that can help reset a person's body clock.

Doctors also encourage teens to make lifestyle changes that promote good sleeping habits. You probably know that caffeine can keep you awake, but many teens don't realize that playing video games or watching TV before sleeping can do the same thing.

night. Some things can trigger more frequent nightmares, including certain medications, drugs, or alcohol. And, ironically, sleep deprivation can also be a cause. The most common triggers for more frequent nightmares, though, are emotional, such as stress or anxiety. If nightmares are interfering with your sleep, it's a good idea to talk to a doctor, therapist, or other counselor.

Sleepwalking

It's rare for teens to walk in their sleep; most sleepwalkers are children. Sleepwalking may run in families. It most often occurs when a person is sick, has a fever, is not getting enough sleep, or is feeling stress.

Because most sleepwalkers don't sleepwalk often, it's not usually a serious problem. Sleepwalkers tend to go back to bed on their own and don't usually remember sleepwalking. (Sleepwalking often happens during the deeper sleep that takes place during stages 3 and 4 of the sleep cycle.) Sometimes, though, a sleepwalker will need help moving around obstacles and getting back to bed. It's also true that waking sleepwalkers can startle them (but it isn't harmful), so try to guide a sleepwalker back to bed gently.

Chapter 18

Insomnia

About Insomnia

What Is Insomnia?

Insomnia, defined as trouble falling asleep or staying asleep, is a common problem. Occasional insomnia is experienced by more than a third of American adults, and chronic insomnia is known to effect more than one in ten. If you have ever suffered from insomnia, you know it can disturb your waking, as well as your sleeping hours. It can cause you to feel sleepy or fatigued during the day, affect your mood, and result in trouble focusing on tasks.

Looking at both the daytime and the nighttime factors of insomnia can help individuals and their healthcare professional understand the causes of this condition, and provide a basis for treating the disorder. Recent research into psychological, lifestyle, environmental, physical and psychiatric factors behind sleep disorders is making it possible for healthcare professionals to help most troubled sleepers.

Types Of Insomnia

Insomnia can occur in people of all ages. Most individuals just experience a night or two of poor sleep, but sometimes the sleep disturbance can last for weeks, months, or even years. Insomnia is most common among women and older adults.

Transient Insomnia: Transient insomnia is the inability to sleep well over a period, lasting fewer than four weeks. This type of insomnia is usually brought on by excitement or stress. Children, for example, may toss and turn just before school starts in the fall, or before an important exam or sporting event. Adults might sleep poorly before an important business meeting or after an argument with a family member or close friend. People are more likely to have trouble sleeping when they are away from home, especially if they have traveled across time zones. Physical activity close to bedtime (within four hours) and illness can also cause this type of insomnia.

Short-Term Insomnia: Short-term insomnia is the inability to sleep well for a period of four weeks to six months. Periods of ongoing stress at work or at home, medical conditions, psychiatric illness, or other persistent factors can result in short-term insomnia. As the cause resolves or the sleeper adjusts to it, sleep will usually return to normal.

Chronic Insomnia: More than 20 million Americans complain of chronic insomnia, defined as poor sleep every night or most nights for more than six months. While most of these individuals worry about their sleep, it's wrong to blame all troubled sleep on worrying. Insomnia may be a physical problem, not due to psychological factors. According to a nationwide study by the Association of Sleep Disorders Centers, physical ailments—such as disorders of breathing or abnormal muscle activity are often the cause of sleep disruption and may account for a large number of self-diagnosed cases of insomnia.

Causes Of Insomnia

What Causes Insomnia?

Insomnia may be independent of other healthcare problems. However, it also may be a symptom of another problem, much like a fever or a stomachache. It can be caused by a number of factors.

Psychological Factors

Vulnerability To Insomnia: Some people seem more likely than others to experience insomnia, just as some people tend to get headaches or upset stomachs. Simply knowing that you may experience insomnia and that it will not last too long can be helpful in dealing with it when it occurs.

Persistent Stress: Exposure to stress may contribute to the development or worsening of insomnia. Relationship problems, a chronically ill child, or an unrewarding career may contribute to sleep problems. If you suffer from these types of stresses, you should seek counseling to gain a new outlook on your troubles and more control in your life.

Learned Insomnia (also known as psychophysiological insomnia): If you sleep poorly, you may worry about not being able to function well during the day. You may try harder to sleep at night, but unfortunately this determined effort can make you more alert, set off a new round of worried thoughts, and cause more sleep loss. Doing activities in and around the bedroom—changing into your night clothes, turning off the lights, pulling up the blankets—can become linked with the sleep problems that follow. Through repetition these bedtime activities can then trigger over-arousal and insomnia. Some individuals with learned insomnia have trouble sleeping in their own beds yet may fall asleep quickly when they don't intend to—while reading the newspaper, sleeping away from home, or watching TV. Just a few nights of poor sleep during a month can be enough to produce a cycle of poor sleep and increase your worry about it. Treatment for learned insomnia aims to improve sleep habits and reduce unnecessary worry.

Lifestyle Factors

Use Of Stimulants: Caffeine near bedtime, even when it doesn't interfere with falling asleep, can trigger awakenings later in the night. Nicotine is also a stimulant, and smokers may take longer to fall asleep than non-smokers. Be aware that the ingredients in many common drugs, including nonprescription drugs for weight loss, asthma, and colds, can disrupt sleep.

Use Of Alcohol: A glass of wine may help you fall asleep quickly, however, alcohol consumption is likely to produce interrupted sleep beginning a few hours after falling asleep.

Erratic Hours: If you do shift work (work non-traditional hours, such as nights or rotating shifts), or maintain later hours on weekends than during the week, you are more likely to experience sleep problems. Maintaining regular hours can help program your body to sleep at certain times and to stay awake at others. Establishing a routine is important.

Environmental Factors

✦ It's A Fact!!
Inactive Behavior: People whose lifestyles are very quiet or restricted may experience difficulty sleeping at night.

Noise: Traffic, airplanes, television, and other noises can disturb sleep even when they don't cause the individual to wake up.

Light: Exposure to bright light prior to sleep can delay sleep onset, while light entering the bedroom can shorten sleep.

All of these environmental factors should be considered if you find yourself feeling tired, even when you think you slept soundly all night.

Illness And Secondary Insomnia

Other sleep disorders, psychiatric and physical illnesses may disrupt sleep, and produce symptoms that can easily be mistaken for insomnia. These other disorders require medical attention and common treatments for insomnia alone will not help.

When insomnia is caused by a psychiatric disorder (most often depression) or a medical disorder (most often chronic pain), it is termed secondary insomnia. Secondary insomnia may be relieved by successful treatment of the primary psychiatric/medical disorder. Additionally, behavioral methods (link) that target the sleep disturbance itself and may quite beneficial especially if some sleep disruption remains after effective treatment of the underlying disorder.

Psychiatric Problems: Insomnia, especially with awakenings earlier than desired, is one of the most frequently reported symptoms of depression. Insomnia is also associated with anxiety disorders, post-traumatic stress disorders, and other conditions. Treatment of the underlying disorder, often including both medication and psychotherapy, can help improve your sleep.

However, additional and specific treatment for the insomnia often is warranted.

Medical Problems: Medical illnesses can disrupt sleep and produce symptoms of insomnia. For example, arthritis, headaches, benign prostatic hypertrophy, and other conditions can cause or worsen the problem of insomnia. Such medical problems usually require the attention of a physician who can diagnose and treat the underlying condition. Treatment of the underlying cause will result in improved sleep. However, in some cases specific treatment for insomnia also will be needed.

Sleep-Related Breathing Disorders: Sleep-related breathing disorders such as sleep apnea can cause repeated pauses in breathing during sleep. This can wake a sleeper dozens or even hundreds of times during the night. Pauses in breathing can be as short as 10 seconds and may not be remembered in the morning. However, they are sufficient to produce disturbed and restless sleep. Severely disrupted breathing during sleep may affect people who breathe normally while they are awake. Breathing-related sleep problems are most common in men, snorers, overweight people, and older adults. Loud snoring that is interrupted by gasps, snorts, or other unusual sounds may be a warning sign of a sleep-related breathing disorder.

✤ It's A Fact!!

Severe cases of sleep apnea often benefit from a treatment known as positive airway pressure (PAP). This treatment involves wearing a mask over the nose during sleep that is connected by a tube to a machine that blows room air into the nose to keep the airway open with a steady stream of air flowing through a mask worn over the nose and mouth during sleep. Other treatments, such as weight loss, surgery, or the use of dental appliances may help some individuals to improve breathing during sleep.

Sleep-Related Periodic Leg Movements: Brief muscle contractions can cause leg jerks that last a second or two and occur repeatedly about every 20–40 seconds for varying periods of time throughout the night (often for an hour or longer). In almost all cases the individual is totally unaware of the limb movements. These movements can cause hundreds of brief interruptions of sleep each night, resulting in restless or non-restorative sleep. Periodic limb movements become more frequent and severe as we grow older. Treatment can include medication, discontinuing medication, evening exercise, a warm bath, elimination of caffeine, or a combination of these. Iron replacement may be helpful if there is an iron deficiency, especially if restless legs syndrome is also present.

Waking Brain Activity: Waking brain activity can persist during sleep. Sleep monitoring during the night has shown that some people who complain of light or less restful sleep show waking brain (EEG) activity occurring simultaneously with sleep activity. Individuals with persistent pain may experience this non-restorative type of sleep.

Gastroesophageal Reflux: Back-up of stomach contents into the esophagus can awaken a person several times a night. This reflux is commonly known as heartburn because of the pain or tightness it produces in the mid-chest area. When reflux occurs during the day, a few swallows and an upright position will usually clear the irritating materials from the esophagus. During sleep, less-frequent swallowing and a lying-down position causes more reflux, making the sleeper wake up coughing and choking. Elevating the head, or raising the head of the bed (headboard) onto 6- to 8-inch blocks may help. Medications can also provide relief.

Next Steps

If you experience recurrent problems with insomnia and it interferes with the way you feel or function during the day, see your healthcare professional or ask for a referral to a sleep disorders specialist. An effective treatment approach may require evaluation of diverse areas such as your psychological state, stress level, activities of daily living, and sleep schedule. Your medical history, a physical exam, and some blood tests may help identify certain causes of the sleep problem.

Insomnia can often be helped through education and information. Some people naturally sleep less than others, and merely need to give up the idea that everyone needs eight hours of sleep. Counseling can help people whose insomnia stems from poor sleep habits. In other cases, medication or evaluation at a sleep disorders center may be recommended.

If you are advised to get an evaluation at a sleep disorders center, you may be asked to keep a sleep diary showing sleeping and waking patterns for a week or two. If you have an appointment at a sleep center, you can expect a physical and psychological examination.

Guidelines For Better Sleep

The following guidelines can be used for a variety of sleep disorders. They may help many people sleep better. For more specific guidelines for your particular sleep disorder, consult your healthcare professional.

- Maintain a regular wake time, even on days off work and on weekends.

- Try to go to bed only when you are drowsy.

- Use your bedroom only for sleep and sex.

- Avoid napping during the daytime. If an occasional nap is necessary, it should be kept to one hour and taken before 3 P.M. The bedroom should be dark, quiet and conducive to sleep.

- Establish a relaxing pre-sleep ritual such as a warm bath, light bedtime snack, or ten minutes of reading.

- Exercise regularly. Mild exercise should not be done within 4 hours of bedtime while vigorous exercise should not be done within 6 hours of bedtime.

- Keep a regular schedule. Regular times for meals, medications, chores, and other activities help keep the inner clock running smoothly.

- Avoid large meals close to bedtime, but a light snack can help promote sound sleep.

✔ Quick Tip

If you are not drowsy and are unable to fall asleep after about 20 minutes in bed, leave your bedroom and engage in a quiet activity elsewhere such as reading a magazine or listening to soft music. Avoid the computer and any stimulating activities. Do not permit yourself to fall asleep outside the bedroom. Return to bed when, and only when, you are sleepy. Repeat this process as often as necessary throughout the night.

- Avoid ingestion of caffeine within six hours of bedtime.

- Teens should avoid alcohol, but people who use alcohol should avoid it especially in the evening. Even a small dose of alcohol can produce dangerous levels of sleepiness if ingested when drowsy.

- Teens should also avoid the use of nicotine, but people who do use nicotine should avoid it especially close to bedtime or during the night.

- Teens should not drink alcohol, and even adults should not drink alcohol while taking sleep medication, sedatives, or other medicines that may interact with alcohol.

Treatment Options

Medication

Sleep medications are recognized as effective and safe treatments for insomnia. Medications that currently are available by prescription are known to improve sleep by reducing the amount of time it takes to fall asleep, increasing sleep duration, or reducing the number of awakenings during sleep. Sleep medications also have been shown to improve self-reports of sleep quality. Sleep medications are often used in conjunction with behavioral treatment of insomnia. Many people who suffer from insomnia find that occasional or short-term use of sleeping pills provides significant relief from their symptoms. Other people may require longer-term use.

While the use of sleep medicines is a common treatment, it is not a cure for insomnia. Sleep medications can be dangerous when treating sleep disruption that may arise from another disorder, such as a sleep-related breathing disorder. Insomnia needs to be properly diagnosed and treatment options discussed with a healthcare professional before treatment with medications is undertaken.

Prescription: There are several types of prescription sleeping pills that have been approved for the treatment of insomnia. These include medications in the class known as benzodiazepines, such as temazepam (Restoril), newer medications that are known as benzodiazepine receptor agonists, such as zolpidem (Ambien) and zaleplon (Sonata). Some may be short-acting and work best for trouble initially falling asleep. Others may be long-acting and work best for maintaining sleep during the night.

✔ Quick Tip

For more information about medications, refer to the American Insomnia Association's section on medication that is available online at http://www.americaninsomniaassociation.org/medications.asp.

Over-The-Counter: Over-the-counter medications are available for the treatment of insomnia. These medications are mainly sedating antihistamines. Such medications certainly may be useful for some individuals, but others find that they are not effective, and are associated with unwanted side effects or lose their effectiveness over time.

Behavioral Treatments

Insomnia is a very common and significant health problem resulting from a variety of causes. Often, misconceptions and worry about sleep, as well as many sleep-disruptive habits, serve important roles in causing and maintaining insomnia problems. When this is the case, behavioral therapies designed to address these causes are often required to eliminate the sleep difficulties. The nature of these treatments varies significantly. Some are composed of fairly formalized "exercises" designed primarily to reduce anxiety and tension at bedtime, whereas others are fairly regimented programs designed to eliminate sleep-disruptive habits. There are several behavioral treatments that are effective and commonly used to treat insomnia.

Relaxation Therapies: Since the late 1950's, a host of formal relaxation therapies, including progressive muscle relaxation training, imagery training, biofeedback, and hypnosis have all been used to treat insomnia. These approaches are designed to reduce anxiety and excessive tension at bedtime. Regardless of the specific relaxation strategy employed, treatment entails teaching the insomnia sufferer a formal exercise or set of exercises designed to reduce anxiety and arousal at bedtime, so that going to sleep becomes less of a problem. Typically, multiple weekly or biweekly treatment sessions are required to teach relaxation skills, which the patient is encouraged to practice

♣ **It's A Fact!!**

Sleep medications may also help with the following conditions:

- **Jet Lag:** A change of several hours in sleep and wake times can trigger both insomnia and daytime sleepiness. For one to three nights, while the body adjusts to time zone changes, taking a sleeping pill may improve sleep and minimize daytime fatigue.

- **Shift Work:** Schedule changes can affect sleep time. Shift workers sometimes find sleeping pills make it easier to fall asleep and stay asleep for one to three nights during a shift change.

- **Acute Stress:** Sleeping pills may prevent persistent sleep problems by helping people prone to insomnia through stressful times, such as a death in the family or the start of a new job.

- **Predictable Stress:** People who always toss and turn the night before a monthly sales meeting or before giving a speech may rest better by taking a sleeping pill at such times.

- **Chronic Insomnia:** Having sleep medications on hand can help ease poor sleepers through periodic flare-ups and reduce the worry that goes along with sleeplessness.

at home in order to gain mastery. The goal of all such treatments is to assist the insomnia sufferer in gaining sufficient relaxation skills in order to reduce anxiety and tension at bedtime to be able to fall asleep.

Stimulus Control: This approach, introduced by Richard Bootzin in 1972, is based on the assumption that both the timing (bedtime) and setting (bed/bedroom) associated with repeated unsuccessful sleep attempts, over time become cues that maintain the insomnia. As a result, the goal of this treatment is to re-associate the bed and bedroom with successful sleep attempts. Stimulus control achieves this by curtailing sleep-incompatible activities in the bed and bedroom and by establishing a consistent sleep-wake schedule. In practice, stimulus control requires that insomnia sufferers:

- go to bed only when sleepy,

- establish a standard wake-up time,

- get out of bed whenever awake for more than 15–20 minutes,

- avoid reading, watching TV, eating, worrying, and other sleep-incompatible behaviors in the bed and bedroom, and

- refrain from daytime napping.

From a practical viewpoint, this treatment has appeal since it is easily understood and can usually be administered in one visit. However, follow-up visits are generally conducted to help the insomnia sufferer achieve optimal success.

Sleep Restriction: Sleep restriction therapy (SRT) is a treatment that aims to reduce the time in bed so that the sleep period follows the individuals biological sleep requirement. This treatment, first introduced by Arthur Spielman and colleagues in 1987, grew out of the observation that many people with insomnia stay in bed hoping this will produce more sleep time. Instead, excess time in bed spreads sleep over a longer period, breaks up sleep, and increases frustration. Typically this treatment begins by having the individual maintain a sleep log to record each night of sleep. After they have maintained a sleep record for about two weeks, the average total sleep time (ATST) is calculated from the information recorded. Using this information, the individual is instructed to stay in bed no longer than ATST + 30 minutes. The time in bed (TIB) is increased by 15–20 minute increments following weeks during which the individual sleeps relatively well but continues to report daytime sleepiness. Conversely, TIB is usually reduced by similar increments following weeks during which the individual continues to have difficulty sleeping. Since TIB adjustments are usually necessary, this therapy typically requires an initial office visit to introduce treatment instructions and follow-up visits to alter TIB instructions.

Cognitive-Behavioral Therapy: This treatment strategy evolved from the above described strategies. Cognitive-Behavioral Insomnia Therapy, or CBT, typically consists of some form of therapy to eliminate the misconceptions and faulty beliefs about sleep that many insomnia sufferers have. For example, it would not be useful for a person who needs only 6½ hours of sleep each night to believe that everyone should try to get 8 hours of sleep on a nightly basis. For such an individual, cognitive therapy designed to challenge this faulty belief often proves useful. In CBT, such cognitive therapy strategies are used in combination with both stimulus control and sleep restriction therapies. One advantage of this treatment is that it includes treatment components which address the range of cognitive and behavioral factors that perpetuate insomnia. As a result, this treatment may be more universally effective across insomnia sufferers regardless of their presenting complaints (for example, sleep onset complaints vs. sleep maintenance difficulty). Admittedly, CBT is a multi-component and seemingly more complex treatment than those previously described. Nonetheless, in practice, this intervention usually requires no more office visits than do the less complex first generation treatments reviewed above. Often, CBT's cognitive therapy and behavioral instructions can be provided in four sessions.

Where To Get Behavioral Treatment For Insomnia

Healthcare practitioners who offer behavioral treatment for insomnia usually have specialized training in the field of sleep medicine, and many are board certified sleep specialists. You can locate a therapist in your area by contacting your local sleep center.

Chapter 19

Delayed Sleep Phase Syndrome

What is delayed sleep phase syndrome?

Delayed sleep phase syndrome, often referred to as DSPS, is a disorder in with the person's sleep-wake cycle (internal clock) is delayed by two or more hours. Basically, it is a shift of the internal clock by two or more hours, in that sleep is postponed. For example, rather than falling asleep at 10:00 P.M. and waking at 7:00 A.M., an adolescent with delayed sleep phase syndrome will not fall asleep until 12:00 A.M. and then has great difficulty awakening at 7:00 A.M. for school or work. If the adolescent is allowed to sleep until late in the morning, he or she will feel rested and can function well. Most adolescents with delayed sleep phase syndrome describe themselves as "night owls" and usually feel and function their best in the evening and nighttime hours. They usually get much less sleep on weekdays compared to weekends or holidays.

Having delayed sleep phase syndrome, especially for adolescents who attend school, can cause significant problems, as they are unable to get up for school, often resulting in multiple school absences and tardiness.

What causes delayed sleep phase syndrome?

Delayed sleep phase syndrome usually develops during adolescence, but can start in childhood. It seldom occurs after the age of 30. Although the cause of delayed sleep phase syndrome is not completely known, it likely is an exaggerated reaction to the normal shift in sleep times that occurs during adolescence. All adolescents have a shift in their internal clock after puberty of about two hours. In those with delayed sleep phase syndrome, the clock shifts even more. In addition, for children who already had a tendency to go to bed late, this normal two-hour shift will result in a significantly shifted internal clock. It is important to realize that this shift in sleep is not caused by deliberate behavior. Unfortunately, many adolescents with delayed sleep phase syndrome get labeled as noncompliant and truants. Approximately 7% of adolescents have delayed sleep phase syndrome, and thus it is a common disorder.

What are the symptoms of delayed sleep phase syndrome?

An adolescent with delayed sleep phase syndrome often experiences the following symptoms.

Daytime Sleepiness: Because of the late sleep onset times, and the usual requirement to get up earlier than desired for school or a job, adolescents with delayed sleep phase syndrome often experience daytime sleepiness as the result of not getting enough sleep.

Inability To Fall Asleep At The Desired Time: On nights that adolescents with delayed sleep phase syndrome try to go to sleep at a "normal" time, they are unable to do so. However, if they were to go to bed at their usual fall asleep time, they would have no problem falling asleep.

Inability To Wake Up At The Desired Time: As a result of the late sleep onset time; many adolescents with delayed sleep phase syndrome are unable to wake up in the morning for school or other activities. This can result in many missed days or being late for school.

> ✤ **It's A Fact!!**
> *How is delayed sleep phase syndrome diagnosed?*
>
> There is no definitive test for delayed sleep phase syndrome so diagnosis is made based on the description of the problem. An overnight sleep study may be recommended to be sure that no other sleep disorder is present, such as obstructive sleep apnea or restless legs syndrome.

No Other Sleep Complaints: Because the internal clock is simply shifted in adolescents with delayed sleep phase syndrome, once asleep they sleep well with few or no awakenings. In addition, on days that they are able to sleep as long as they wish, especially on weekends or holidays, sleep is normal and daytime sleepiness is not experienced.

Other Daytime Symptoms: Some adolescents with delayed sleep phase syndrome experience problems with depression and other behavior problems as a result of the daytime sleepiness and the effects of missing school and social activities. In addition, there are a percentage of adolescents with delayed sleep phase syndrome who have school refusal, which complicates both diagnosis and treatment.

How is delayed sleep phase syndrome treated?

Delayed sleep phase syndrome is a difficult disorder to treat and requires significant effort on the part of the adolescent. Thus, for treatment to be successful, the adolescent has to be very motivated. The goal of treatment is to re-train the internal clock to a more regular schedule. Making the initial shift in the sleep-wake cycle is easier, however, than maintaining that change. Treatment can involve the following:

Sleep Hygiene: Good sleep habits are especially important for adolescents with delayed sleep phase syndrome. These habits should include a regular sleep schedule that includes going to bed and waking up at the same time every day; avoidance of caffeine, smoking, and other drugs; a bedroom environment that is cool, quiet, and comfortable; a bedtime routine that is calm and sleep-inducing; and avoidance of all stimulating activities before bed, such as computer games and television.

Shifting The Internal Clock: Treatment for delayed sleep phase syndrome involves systematically advancing or delaying bedtime on successive nights.

- *Phase advancement:* Phase advancement involves moving the bedtime earlier by 15 minutes on successive nights. If the adolescent usually falls asleep at 12:30, then bedtime is set for 12:15 for one or two nights, 12:00 for one to two nights, and so on.

- *Phase delay (chronotherapy):* Phase delay is chosen if the adolescent's naturally occurring bedtime is three or more hours later than desired. Bedtime is delayed by two to three hours on successive nights. For example, if an adolescent usually falls asleep at 2:00 A.M., bedtime is delayed until 4:00 A.M. on night one, 6:00 A.M. on night two, and so on until the desired bedtime is reached (for example, 10:30 P.M.). Given that it is much easier for the body to adjust to a later bedtime than an earlier one, it is often recommended to delay bedtime rather than try to advance it.

- *Sticking with it:* Once the desired bedtime is reached, the adolescent must stick with it on a nightly basis. Even one night of late night studying or socializing can return the internal clock to being delayed. Usually, however, after several months, the schedule can become a bit more flexible.

Bright Light Therapy: Sometimes bright light therapy is recommended which involves exposure to bright light in the morning for approximately 20–30 minutes, and avoidance of bright light in the evening. Bright light in the morning will help reset the body's internal clock. Special light boxes need to be purchased for this treatment.

Chapter 20

Snoring

UUGHGHGHGHHHSSHHH!! UUGHGHGHGHHHSSHHH!!

There's nothing worse than the sound of someone snoring if you're trying to fall asleep. Or maybe it's you who snores, and people tease you about the noise you make in your sleep. Snoring isn't just noisy. Sometimes it's a sign of a serious problem that should be treated by a doctor. Read on to find out more about the snore!

Snoozing Or Snoring?

Snoring is a fairly common problem that can happen to anyone—young or old. Snoring happens when a person can't move air freely through his or her nose and mouth during sleep. That annoying sound is caused by certain structures in the mouth and throat—the tongue, upper throat, soft palate (say: pa-lut), uvula (say: yoo-vyuh-luh), as well as big tonsils and adenoids—vibrating against each other.

What Makes You Snore?

There are many reasons why people snore. Here are some of the most common:

About This Chapter: This information was provided by TeensHealth, one of the largest resources online for medically reviewed health information written for parents, kids, and teens. For more articles like this one, visit www.TeensHealth.org, or www.KidsHealth.org. © 2004 The Nemours Foundation.

- Seasonal allergies can make some people's noses stuffy and cause them to snore.

- Blocked nasal passages or airways (due to a cold or sinus infection) can cause a rattling snore.

- A deviated septum, which is the tissue and cartilage that separates the two nostrils in your nose, may be crooked. Some people with a very deviated septum have surgery to straighten it out. This also helps them breathe better—not just stop snoring.

♣ **It's A Fact!!**
People usually find out they snore from the people who live with them. Kids may find out they snore from a brother or sister or from a friend who sleeps over. Snoring keeps other people awake and probably doesn't let the snoring person get top quality rest, either.

- Enlarged or swollen tonsils or adenoids may cause a person to snore. Tonsils and adenoids (adenoids are glands located inside of your head, near the inner parts of your nasal passages) help trap harmful bacteria, but they can become very big and swollen all of the time. Many kids who snore have this problem.

- Drinking alcohol can relax the tongue and throat muscles too much, which partially blocks air movement as someone is breathing and can contribute to snoring noises.

- Being overweight can cause narrowing of the air passages. Many people who are very overweight snore.

Snoring is also one symptom of a serious sleep disorder known as sleep apnea. When a person has sleep apnea, his or her breathing is irregular during sleep. Typically, a person with sleep apnea will actually stop breathing for short amounts of time 30 to 300 times a night! It can be a big problem if the person doesn't get enough oxygen.

People with this disorder often wake up with bad headaches and feel exhausted all day long. They may be very drowsy and have difficulty staying awake while having a conversation or even while driving. Kids affected by sleep apnea may be irritable and have difficulty concentrating, particularly in school and with homework.

Snoring Solutions

According to the government's patent office (this is where you go to register an idea or invention), there are hundreds of anti-snoring devices on the market. Some of them startle you awake when they sense you are snoring. Unfortunately, they may only work because they keep you awake.

Those small, white strips some football players wear across their noses that kind of look like a bandage are another anti-snoring device. Football players wear them during the game to breathe easier while running a play or making a tackle. People also wear these breathing strips to try to stop snoring.

Other snoring solutions include tilting the top of a bed upward a few inches, changing sleeping positions (from the back to a side), and not eating a heavy meal (or for an adult, not drinking alcohol) before bedtime. These kinds of "cures" may work only for someone who snores occasionally and lightly—or they may not work at all.

If you can't stop snoring or the snoring becomes heavy, it's a good idea to see a doctor. He or she might tell you how to keep your nasal passages clear and will check your tonsils and adenoids to be sure they aren't enlarged and don't have to be removed.

Some people need to lose weight, change their diets, or develop regular sleeping patterns to stop snoring. It may be helpful to remove allergy triggers (stuffed animals, pets, and feather/down pillows and comforters) from the person's bedroom. The doctor might also suggest medications for allergies or congestion due to a cold.

If a doctor suspects a person has sleep apnea, he or she will monitor the patient while they sleep. This is usually done in a sleep center (a medical building that has equipment to monitor breathing during sleep). A patient is attached

☞ Remember!!
Solving a snoring problem lets everyone
breathe and sleep a little easier.

to machines that check heart rate, oxygen and carbon dioxide levels, eye movement, chest wall movement, and the flow of air through the nose.

The doctor can then tell if a patient has a disorder like sleep apnea. The best thing about the test is that it doesn't hurt at all. After all, you sleep right through it. Once doctors know what's wrong, you can be treated for it, usually with lifestyle changes, sometimes medicines, or even surgery, if necessary.

Chapter 21

Sleep Apnea

What is sleep apnea?

Sleep apnea is a common disorder that can be very serious. In sleep apnea, your breathing stops or gets very shallow while you are sleeping. Each pause in breathing typically lasts 10 to 20 seconds or more. These pauses can occur 20 to 30 times or more an hour.

The most common type of sleep apnea is obstructive sleep apnea. During sleep, enough air cannot flow into your lungs through your mouth and nose even though you try to breathe. When this happens, the amount of oxygen in your blood may drop. Normal breaths then start again with a loud snort or choking sound.

When your sleep is upset throughout the night, you can be very sleepy during the day. With sleep apnea, your sleep is not restful because:

- These brief episodes of increased airway resistance (and breathing pauses) occur many times.

- You may have many brief drops in the oxygen levels in your blood.

- You move out of deep sleep and into light sleep several times during the night, resulting in poor sleep quality.

About This Chapter: "Sleep Apnea," National Heart, Lung, and Blood Institute (www.nhlbi.nih.gov), February 2006.

People with sleep apnea often have loud snoring. However, not everyone who snores has sleep apnea. Some people with sleep apnea don't know they snore.

Untreated sleep apnea can increase the chance of having high blood pressure and even a heart attack or stroke. Untreated sleep apnea can also increase the risk of diabetes and the risk for work-related accidents and driving accidents.

> **✔ Quick Tip**
>
> • Sleep apnea happens more often in people who are overweight, but even thin people can have it.
>
> • Most people don't know they have sleep apnea. They don't know that they are having problems breathing while they are sleeping.
>
> • A family member or bed partner may notice the signs of sleep apnea first.

What causes sleep apnea?

Sleep apnea happens when enough air cannot move into your lungs while you are sleeping. When you are awake, and normally during sleep, your throat muscles keep your throat open and air flows into your lungs. In obstructive sleep apnea, however, the throat briefly collapses, causing pauses in your breathing. With pauses in breathing, the oxygen level in your blood may drop. This happens if the following conditions occur:

• Your throat muscles and tongue relax more than is normal.

• Your tonsils and adenoids are large.

• You are overweight. The extra soft tissue in your throat makes it harder to keep the throat area open.

• The shape of your head and neck (bony structure) results in somewhat smaller airway size in the mouth and throat area.

With the throat frequently fully or partly blocked during sleep, enough air cannot flow into your lungs, even though your efforts to breathe continue. Your breathing may become hard and noisy and may even stop for short periods of time (apneas).

Central apnea is a rare type of sleep apnea that happens when the area of your brain that controls your breathing doesn't send the correct signals to the breathing muscles. Then there is no effort to breathe at all for brief periods. Snoring does not typically occur in central apnea.

Who is at risk for obstructive sleep apnea?

Anyone can have obstructive sleep apnea.

It is estimated that more than 12 million Americans have obstructive sleep apnea. More than half the people who have sleep apnea are overweight, and most snore heavily.

Sleep apnea is more common in men. One out of 25 middle-aged men and one out of 50 middle-aged women have sleep apnea that causes them to be very sleepy during the day. Sleep apnea is more common in African Americans, Hispanics, and Pacific Islanders than in Caucasians. If someone in your family has sleep apnea, you are more likely to develop it than someone without a family history of the condition.

Adults who are most likely to have sleep apnea:

- Snore loudly.

- Are overweight.

- Have high blood pressure.

- Have a decreased size of the airways in their nose, throat, or mouth. This can be caused by the shape of these structures or by medical conditions causing congestion in these areas, such as hay fever or other allergies.

- Have a family history of sleep apnea.

✔ **Quick Tip**

Obstructive sleep apnea can also occur in children who snore. If someone you know snores, you should discuss it with them so that they can talk to their doctor or health care provider.

What are the signs and symptoms of sleep apnea?

The most common signs of sleep apnea are:

- Loud snoring

- Choking or gasping during sleep

- Fighting sleepiness during the day (even at work or while driving)

- Your family members may notice the symptoms before you do. Otherwise, you will likely not be aware that you have problems breathing while you are asleep.

Others signs of sleep apnea may include:

- Morning headaches

- Memory or learning problems

- Feeling irritable

- Not being able to concentrate on your work

- Mood swings or personality changes; perhaps feeling depressed

- Dry throat when you wake up

- Frequent urination at night

How is sleep apnea diagnosed?

Your doctor will do a physical exam and take a medical history that includes asking you and your family questions about how you sleep and how you function during the day. As part of the exam, your doctor will check your mouth, nose, and throat for extra or large tissues; for example, tonsils, uvula (the tissue that hangs from the middle of the back of the mouth), and soft palate (the roof of your mouth in the back of your throat).

Your doctor may order a sleep recording of what happens with your breathing while you sleep. A sleep recording is a test that is often done in a sleep center or sleep laboratory, which may be part of a hospital. You may stay overnight in the sleep center, although sleep studies are sometimes done in the home. The most common sleep recording used to find out if you have sleep apnea is called a polysomnogram, or PSG. This test records:

- Brain activity,

- Eye movement,

- Muscle activity,

- Breathing and heart rate,

- How much air moves in and out of your lungs while you are sleeping, and

- The percentage of oxygen in your blood.

A PSG is painless. You will go to sleep as usual. The staff at the sleep center will monitor your sleep throughout the night. The results of your PSG will be analyzed by a sleep medicine specialist to see if you have sleep apnea, how severe it is, and what treatment may be recommended.

In certain circumstances, the PSG can be done at home. A home monitor can be used to record your heart rate, how air moves in and out of your lungs, the amount of oxygen in your blood, and your breathing effort. For this test, a technician will come to your home and help you apply the monitor that you will wear overnight. You will go to sleep as usual, and the technician will come back the next morning to get the monitor and send the results to your doctor.

Once all your tests are completed, the sleep medicine specialist will review the results and work with you and your family to develop a treatment plan. In some cases, you may also need to see another physician for evaluation of:

- Lung problems (treated by a pulmonologist).

- Problems with the brain or nerves (treated by a neurologist).

- Heart or blood pressure problems (treated by a cardiologist).

- Ear, nose, or throat problems (treated by an ENT specialist).

- Mental health, such as anxiety or depression (treated by a psychologist or psychiatrist).

How is sleep apnea treated?

Treatment is aimed at restoring regular nighttime breathing and relieving symptoms such as very loud snoring and daytime sleepiness. Treatment will also help associated medical problems, such as high blood pressure, and reduce the risk for heart attack and stroke.

Changes In Activities Or Habits: If you have mild sleep apnea, some changes in daily activities or habits may be all that are needed:

- Avoid alcohol, smoking, and medicines that make you sleepy. They make it harder for your throat to stay open while you sleep.

- Lose weight if you are overweight. Even a little weight loss can improve your symptoms.

- Sleep on your side instead of your back. Sleeping on your side may help keep your throat open.

People with moderate or severe sleep apnea will need to make these changes as well. They also will need other treatments, such as the following.

Continuous Positive Airway Pressure: Continuous positive airway pressure (CPAP) is the most common treatment for sleep apnea. For this treatment, you wear a mask over your nose during sleep. The mask blows air into your throat at a pressure level that is right for you. The increased airway pressure keeps the throat open while you sleep. The air pressure is adjusted so that it is just enough to stop the airways from briefly getting too small during sleep.

Sleep apnea will return if CPAP is stopped or if it is not used correctly. Usually, a technician comes to your home to bring the CPAP equipment. The technician will set up the CPAP machine and make adjustments based on your doctor's orders.

CPAP treatment may cause side effects in some people. Some side effects are:

- Dry or stuffy nose

- Irritation of the skin on your face

- Bloating of your stomach

- Sore eyes

- Headaches

☞ Remember!!
Treating sleep apnea may help you stop snoring. Stopping snoring does not mean that you no longer have sleep apnea or that you can stop using CPAP.

✎ What's It Mean?

Orthodontist: A specialist in correcting teeth or jaw problems.

If you are having trouble with CPAP side effects, work with your sleep medicine specialist and technician. Together you can do things to reduce these side effects, such as:

- Use a nasal spray to relieve a dry, stuffy, or runny nose.

- Adjust the CPAP settings.

- Adjust the size/fit of the mask.

- Add moisture to the air as it flows through the mask.

- Use a CPAP machine that can automatically adjust the amount of air pressure to the level that is required to keep the airway open.

- Use a CPAP machine that will start with a low air pressure and slowly increase the air pressure as you fall asleep.

People with severe sleep apnea symptoms generally feel much better once they begin treatment with CPAP. When using CPAP, it is very important that you follow up with your doctor. If you are having side effects, talk to your doctor.

Mouthpiece: A mouthpiece (oral appliance) may be helpful in some people with mild sleep apnea. Some doctors may also recommend this if you snore loudly but do not have sleep apnea.

A custom-fit plastic mouthpiece will be made by a dentist or orthodontist. The mouthpiece will adjust your lower jaw and your tongue to help keep the airway in your throat open while you are sleeping. Air can then flow easily into your lungs because there is less resistance to breathing.

Possible side effects of the mouthpiece include damage to your:

- Teeth

- Gums

- Jaw

Follow up with your dentist or orthodontist to check for any side effects and to be sure that your mouthpiece fits.

Surgery: Some people with sleep apnea may benefit from surgery. The type of surgery depends on the cause of the sleep apnea.

- Surgery may be done to remove the tonsils and adenoids if they are blocking the airway. This surgery is especially helpful for children.

- Uvulopalatopharyngoplasty (UPPP) is a surgery that removes the tonsils, uvula (the tissue that hangs from the middle of the back of the roof of the mouth), and part of your soft palate (the roof of your mouth in the back of your throat). This surgery is only effective for some people with sleep apnea.

- Laser-assisted uvulopalatoplasty (LAUP) is a surgery that can stop snoring but is probably not helpful in treating sleep apnea. A laser device is used to remove the uvula and part of the soft palate. Because this surgery stops the main symptom of sleep apnea (snoring), it is important to have a sleep study first.

- Tracheostomy is a surgery used in severe sleep apnea. A small hole is made in the windpipe and a tube is inserted. Air will flow through the tube and into the lungs. This surgery is very successful but is needed only in patients not responding to all other possible treatments.

Other possible surgeries for some people with sleep apnea include:

- Rebuilding the lower jaw

- Surgery on the nose

- Surgery to treat obesity

Currently, there are no medicines for the treatment of sleep apnea.

What's it like living with sleep apnea?

Getting treatment for sleep apnea and following your doctor's advice can help you and your family members.

- Getting treatment for sleep apnea can help snoring and can improve your sleep.

- Treating sleep apnea helps you feel rested during the day.

- Many people will benefit by making healthy changes, such as stopping smoking and losing weight.

- Some people will need to wear a mask at night to help keep the throat open and improve breathing.

- A few people will need to have surgery to remove tonsils and adenoids, part of the uvula and the soft palate that may block the airway.

- Regular and ongoing follow-up is needed; your sleep medicine specialist will check whether your treatment is working and whether you are having any side effects.

What can family do to help?

Often, people with sleep apnea do not know they have it. They are not aware that their breathing stops and starts many times while they are sleeping. Family members or bed partners are usually the first ones to notice that the person snores and stops breathing while sleeping.

There are many things family members can do to help a loved one who has sleep apnea, including:

- Letting the person know if he or she snores loudly during sleep or has breathing stops and starts

- Encouraging the person to get medical help

- Helping the person follow the doctor's treatment plan, including continuous positive airway pressure (CPAP)

- Making sure the person puts on the CPAP mask before falling asleep

- Providing emotional support

- Helping with insurance paperwork

Sleep apnea can be very serious. People with sleep apnea are at higher risk for car crashes, work-related accidents, and other medical problems due to their sleepiness. It is important that people with sleep apnea see their doctor to treat and control this disorder.

Treatment may improve a person's overall health and happiness as well as the quality of sleep for both the person and the entire family.

🖝 Remember!!

- Sleep apnea is a common breathing disorder that can be very serious.

- In sleep apnea, your breathing stops or becomes very shallow for periods of 10 to 20 seconds or longer many times during the night.

- The most common type of sleep apnea is obstructive sleep apnea.

- It is estimated that more than 12 million Americans have sleep apnea.

- The most common signs of sleep apnea are loud snoring and choking or gasping during sleep and being sleepy during the day.

- Having a physical exam and providing your doctor with information about your sleep will help to diagnose sleep apnea. Your doctor may also want you to have special sleep tests.

- Treatment is aimed at restoring regular nighttime breathing and relieving symptoms such as loud snoring and daytime sleepiness. Treatment will also help associated medical problems, such as high blood pressure, and reduce the risk for heart attack and stroke.

- Continuous positive airway pressure (CPAP) is the most common treatment for sleep apnea.

- Some people with sleep apnea may benefit from surgery.

- Family members can help a person who snores loudly or stops breathing while sleeping by encouraging him or her to get medical help.

- Treatment for sleep apnea may improve a person's overall health and happiness as well as the quality of sleep for both the person and the entire family.

Chapter 22

Narcolepsy

What is narcolepsy?

Narcolepsy is a chronic neurological disorder caused by the brain's inability to regulate sleep-wake cycles normally. At various times throughout the day, people with narcolepsy experience fleeting urges to sleep. If the urge becomes overwhelming, patients fall asleep for periods lasting from a few seconds to several minutes. In rare cases, some people may remain asleep for an hour or longer.

Narcoleptic sleep episodes can occur at any time, and thus frequently prove profoundly disabling. People may involuntarily fall asleep while at work or at school, when having a conversation, playing a game, eating a meal, or, most dangerously, when driving an automobile or operating other types of potentially hazardous machinery. In addition to daytime sleepiness, three other major symptoms frequently characterize narcolepsy: cataplexy; vivid hallucinations during sleep onset or upon awakening; and brief episodes of total paralysis at the beginning or end of sleep.

Contrary to common beliefs, people with narcolepsy do not spend a substantially greater proportion of their time asleep during a 24-hour period than do normal sleepers. In addition to daytime drowsiness and involuntary sleep

About This Chapter: "Narcolepsy Fact Sheet," National Institute of Neurological Disorders and Stroke, March 23, 2007.

episodes, most patients also experience frequent awakenings during nighttime sleep. For these reasons, narcolepsy is considered to be a disorder of the normal boundaries between the sleeping and waking states.

For most adults, a normal night's sleep lasts about 8 hours and is composed of four to six separate sleep cycles. A sleep cycle is defined by a segment of non-rapid eye movement (NREM) sleep followed by a period of rapid eye movement (REM) sleep. The NREM segment can be further divided into stages according to the size and frequency of brain waves. REM sleep, in contrast, is accompanied by bursts of rapid eye movement along with sharply heightened brain activity and temporary paralysis of the muscles that control posture and body movement. When subjects are awakened from sleep, they report that they were "having a dream" more often if they had been in REM sleep than if they had been in NREM sleep. Transitions from NREM to REM sleep are governed by interactions among groups of neurons (nerve cells) in certain parts of the brain.

Scientists now believe that narcolepsy results from disease processes affecting brain mechanisms that regulate REM sleep. For normal sleepers a typical sleep cycle is about 100–110 minutes long, beginning with NREM sleep and transitioning to REM sleep after 80–100 minutes. But, people with narcolepsy frequently enter REM sleep within a few minutes of falling asleep.

Who gets narcolepsy?

Narcolepsy is not rare, but it is an under-recognized and under-diagnosed condition. According to current estimates, the disorder affects about one in

---

✎ What's It Mean?

Cataplexy: The sudden loss of voluntary muscle tone.

Obstructive Sleep Apnea: A temporary cessation of breathing that occurs repeatedly during sleep and is caused by a narrowing of the airway.

Restless Legs Syndrome: A neurological disorder characterized by unpleasant sensations—burning, creeping, tugging—in the legs and an uncontrollable urge to move when at rest.

Source: National Institute of Neurological Disorders and Stroke, 2007.

every 2,000 Americans—a total of more than 135,000 individuals. After obstructive sleep apnea and restless legs syndrome, narcolepsy is the third most frequently diagnosed primary sleep disorder found in patients seeking treatment at sleep clinics. But the exact prevalence rate remains uncertain, and the disorder may affect a larger segment of the population than currently estimated.

Narcolepsy appears throughout the world in every racial and ethnic group, affecting males and females equally. But prevalence rates vary among populations. Compared to the U.S. population, for example, the prevalence rate is substantially lower in Israel (about one per 500,000) and considerably higher in Japan (about one per 600).

Most cases of narcolepsy are sporadic—that is, the disorder occurs independently in individuals without strong evidence of being inherited. But familial clusters are known to occur. Up to 10 percent of patients diagnosed with narcolepsy with cataplexy report having a close relative with the same symptoms. Genetic factors alone are not sufficient to cause narcolepsy. Other factors—such as infection, immune-system dysfunction, trauma, hormonal changes, stress—may also be present before the disease develops. Thus, while close relatives of people with narcolepsy have a statistically higher risk of developing the disorder than do members of the general population, that risk remains low in comparison to diseases that are purely genetic in origin.

What are the symptoms?

People with narcolepsy experience highly individualized patterns of REM sleep disturbances that tend to begin subtly and may change dramatically over time. The most common major symptom, other than excessive daytime sleepiness (EDS), is cataplexy, which occurs in about 70 percent of all patients. Sleep paralysis and hallucinations are somewhat less common. Only 10 to 25 percent of patients, however, display all four of these major symptoms during the course of their illness.

Excessive Daytime Sleepiness: EDS, the symptom most consistently experienced by almost all patients, is usually the first to become clinically apparent. Generally, EDS interferes with normal activities on a daily basis, whether or not patients have sufficient sleep at night. People with

EDS describe it as a persistent sense of mental cloudiness, a lack of energy, a depressed mood, or extreme exhaustion. Many find that they have great difficulty maintaining their concentration while at school or work. Some experience memory lapses. Many find it nearly impossible to stay alert in passive situations, as when listening to lectures or watching television. People tend to awaken from such unavoidable sleeps feeling refreshed and finding that their feelings of drowsiness and fatigue subside for an hour or two.

Involuntary sleep episodes are sometimes very brief, lasting no more than seconds at a time. As many as 40 percent of all people with narcolepsy are prone to automatic behavior during such "microsleeps." They fall asleep for a few seconds while performing a task but continue carrying it through to completion without any apparent interruption. During these episodes, people are usually engaged in habitual, essentially "second nature" activities such as taking notes in class, typing, or driving. They cannot recall their actions, and their performance is almost always impaired during a microsleep. Their handwriting may, for example, degenerate into an illegible scrawl, or they may store items in bizarre locations and then forget where they placed them. If an episode occurs while driving, patients may get lost or have an accident.

Cataplexy: Cataplexy is a sudden loss of muscle tone that leads to feelings of weakness and a loss of voluntary muscle control. Attacks can occur at any time during the waking period, with patients usually experiencing their first episodes several weeks or months after the onset of EDS. But in about 10 percent of all cases, cataplexy is the first symptom to appear and can be misdiagnosed as a manifestation of a seizure disorder. Cataplectic attacks vary in duration and severity. The loss of muscle tone can be barely perceptible, involving no more than a momentary sense of slight weakness in a limited number of muscles, such as mild drooping of the eyelids. The most severe attacks result in a complete loss of tone in all voluntary muscles, leading to total physical collapse in which patients are unable to move, speak, or keep their eyes open. But even during the most severe episodes, people remain fully conscious, a characteristic that distinguishes cataplexy from seizure disorders. Although cataplexy can occur spontaneously, it is more often triggered by sudden, strong emotions such as fear, anger, stress, excitement, or humor. Laughter is reportedly the most frequent trigger.

The loss of muscle tone during a cataplectic episode resembles the interruption of muscle activity that naturally occurs during REM sleep. A group of neurons in the brainstem ceases activity during REM sleep, inhibiting muscle movement. Using an animal model, scientists have recently learned that this same group of neurons becomes inactive during cataplectic attacks, a discovery that provides a clue to at least one of the neurological abnormalities contributing to human narcoleptic symptoms.

Sleep Paralysis: The temporary inability to move or speak while falling asleep or waking up also parallels REM-induced inhibitions of voluntary muscle activity. This natural inhibition usually goes unnoticed by people who experience normal sleep because it occurs only when they are fully asleep and entering the REM stage at the appropriate time in the sleep cycle. Experiencing sleep paralysis resembles undergoing a cataplectic attack affecting the entire body. As with cataplexy, people remain fully conscious. Cataplexy and sleep paralysis are frightening events, especially when first experienced. Shocked by suddenly being unable to move, many patients fear that they may be permanently paralyzed or even dying. However, even when severe, cataplexy and sleep paralysis do not result in permanent dysfunction. After episodes end, people rapidly recover their full capacity to move and speak.

Hallucinations: Hallucinations can accompany sleep paralysis or can occur in isolation when people are falling asleep or waking up. Referred to as hypnagogic hallucinations when accompanying sleep onset and as hypnopompic hallucinations when occurring during awakening, these delusional experiences are unusually vivid and frequently frightening. Most often, the content is primarily visual, but any of the other senses can be involved. These hallucinations represent another intrusion of an element of REM sleep—dreaming—into the wakeful state.

When do symptoms appear?

In most cases, symptoms first appear when people are between the ages of 10 and 25 but narcolepsy can become clinically apparent at virtually any age. Many patients first experience symptoms between the ages of 35 and

45. A smaller number initially manifest the disorder around the ages of 50 to 55. Narcolepsy can also develop early in life, probably more frequently than is generally recognized. For example, 3-year-old children have been diagnosed with the disorder. Whatever the age of onset, patients find that the symptoms tend to get worse over the two to three decades after the first symptoms appear. Many older patients find that some daytime symptoms decrease in severity after age 60.

Narcoleptic symptoms, especially EDS, often prove more severe when the disorder develops early in life rather than during the adult years. Experts have also begun to recognize that narcolepsy sometimes contributes to certain childhood behavioral problems, such as attention deficit hyperactivity disorder, and must be addressed before the behavioral problem can be resolved. If left undiagnosed and untreated, narcolepsy can pose special problems for children and adolescents, interfering with their psychological, social, and cognitive development and undermining their ability to succeed at school. For some young people, feelings of low self-esteem due to poor academic performance may persist into adulthood.

What causes narcolepsy?

The cause of narcolepsy remains unknown but during the past decade, scientists have made considerable progress in understanding its pathogenesis and in identifying genes strongly associated with the disorder. Researchers have also discovered abnormalities in various parts of the brain involved in regulating REM sleep that appear to contribute to symptom development. Experts now believe it is likely that—similar to many other complex, chronic neurological diseases—narcolepsy involves multiple factors interacting to cause neurological dysfunction and REM sleep disturbances.

A number of variant forms (alleles) of genes located in a region of chromosome 6 known as the HLA complex have proved to be strongly, although not invariably, associated with narcolepsy. The HLA complex comprises a large number of interrelated genes that regulate key aspects of immune-system function. The majority of people diagnosed with narcolepsy are known to have specific variants in certain HLA genes. However, these variations are neither necessary nor sufficient to cause the disorder. Some people with narcolepsy do not have the variant genes, while many people in the general population without narcolepsy do possess these variant genes. Thus it appears that specific variations in HLA genes increase an individual's predisposition to develop the disorder—possibly through a yet-undiscovered route involving changes in immune-system function—when other causative factors are present.

Many other genes besides those making up the HLA complex may contribute to the development of narcolepsy. Groups of neurons in several parts of the brainstem and the central brain, including the thalamus and hypothalamus, interact to control sleep. Large numbers of genes on different chromosomes control these neurons' activities, any of which could contribute to development of the disease. Scientists studying narcolepsy in dogs have identified a mutation in a gene on chromosome 12 that appears to contribute to the disorder. This mutated gene disrupts the processing of a special class of neurotransmitters called hypocretins (also known as Orexins) that are produced by neurons located in the hypothalamus. The neurons that produce hypocretins are active during wakefulness, and research suggests that they keep the brain systems needed for wakefulness from shutting down unexpectedly. Mice born without functioning hypocretin genes develop many symptoms of narcolepsy.

✎ What's It Mean?

Neurotransmitters: Special proteins that neurons produce to communicate with each other and to regulate biological processes.

Source: National Institute of Neurological Disorders and Stroke, 2007.

Except in rare cases, narcolepsy in humans is not associated with mutations of the hypocretin gene. However, scientists have found that brains from humans with narcolepsy often contain greatly reduced numbers of hypocretin-producing neurons. Certain HLA subtypes may increase susceptibility to an immune attack on hypocretin neurons in the hypothalamus, leading to degeneration of neurons in the hypocretin system. Other factors also may interfere with proper functioning of this system. The hypocretins regulate appetite and feeding behavior in addition to controlling sleep. Therefore, the loss of hypocretin-producing neurons may explain not only how narcolepsy develops in some people, but also why people with narcolepsy have higher rates of obesity compared to the general population.

Other factors appear to play important roles in the development of narcolepsy. Some rare cases are known to result from traumatic injuries to parts of the brain involved in REM sleep or from tumor growth and other disease processes in the same regions. Infections, exposure to toxins, dietary factors, stress, hormonal changes such as those occurring during puberty or menopause, and alterations in a person's sleep schedule are just a few of the many factors that may exert direct or indirect effects on the brain, thereby possibly contributing to disease development.

How is narcolepsy diagnosed?

Narcolepsy is not definitively diagnosed in most patients until 10 to 15 years after the first symptoms appear. This unusually long lag-time is due to several factors, including the disorder's subtle onset and the variability of symptoms. As important, however, is the fact that the public is largely unfamiliar with the disorder, as are many health professionals. When symptoms initially develop, people often do not recognize that they are experiencing the onset of a distinct neurological disorder and thus fail to seek medical treatment.

A clinical examination and exhaustive medical history are essential for diagnosis and treatment. However, none of the major symptoms is exclusive to narcolepsy. EDS can result from a wide range of medical conditions, including other sleep disorders such as sleep apnea, various viral or bacterial infections, mood disorders such as depression, and painful chronic illnesses such as congestive heart failure and rheumatoid arthritis that disrupt normal sleep patterns. Various medications can also lead to EDS, as can consumption of caffeine, alcohol, and nicotine. Finally, sleep deprivation has become one of the most common causes of EDS among Americans.

This lack of specificity greatly increases the difficulty of arriving at an accurate diagnosis based on a consideration of symptoms alone. Thus, a battery of specialized tests, which can be performed in a sleep disorders clinic, is usually required before a diagnosis can be established.

♣ It's A Fact!!
Tests Used To Diagnose Narcolepsy

Sleep tests are usually done at a sleep disorders center. For some sleep tests, you may need to sleep overnight at the center. Other sleep tests can be done during the day. The three tests most often used to diagnose narcolepsy are:

• Polysomnogram (PSG)

• Multiple sleep latency test (MSLT)

• Hypocretin test

Polysomnogram: For this study, you sleep overnight at a sleep center. While you are sleeping, the staff at the center use various devices to measure your brain activity, breathing, and movements. The signs of narcolepsy this test can reveal include:

• Falling asleep quickly

• Entering rapid eye movement (REM) sleep soon after falling asleep

• Waking up often during the night

Multiple Sleep Latency Test: This test is usually done during the day after an overnight PSG. Also called a nap study, the MSLT measures how easy it is for you to fall asleep during the day. You are asked to take short naps about every 2 hours. The test records eye movements, muscle tone, and brain activity with small devices attached to the head. The signs of narcolepsy this test can reveal are quickly falling asleep during the day (after a full night's sleep) and entering REM sleep soon after falling asleep.

Hypocretin Test: This test measures the levels of hypocretin in the fluid that bathes your spinal cord. Low levels of hypocretin make it likely that you have narcolepsy.

Source: Excerpted from "Narcolepsy," National Heart, Lung, and Blood Institute, 2006.

What treatments are available?

Narcolepsy cannot yet be cured. But EDS and cataplexy, the most disabling symptoms of the disorder, can be controlled in most patients with drug treatment. Often the treatment regimen is modified as symptoms change.

For decades, doctors have used central nervous system stimulants—amphetamines such as methylphenidate, dextroamphetamine, methamphetamine, and pemoline—to alleviate EDS and reduce the incidence of sleep attacks. For most patients these medications are generally quite effective at reducing daytime drowsiness and improving levels of alertness. However, they are associated with a wide array of undesirable side effects so their use must be carefully monitored. Common side effects include irritability and nervousness, shakiness, disturbances in heart rhythm, stomach upset, nighttime sleep disruption, and anorexia. Patients may also develop tolerance with long-term use, leading to the need for increased dosages to maintain effectiveness. In addition, doctors should be careful when prescribing these drugs and patients should be careful using them because the potential for abuse is high with any amphetamine.

In 1999, the FDA approved a new non-amphetamine wake-promoting drug called modafinil for the treatment of EDS. In clinical trials, modafinil proved to be effective in alleviating EDS while producing fewer, less serious side effects that do amphetamines. Headache is the most commonly reported adverse effect. Long-term use of modafinil does not appear to lead to tolerance.

Two classes of antidepressant drugs have proved effective in controlling cataplexy in many patients: tricyclics (including imipramine, desipramine, clomipramine, and protriptyline) and selective serotonin reuptake inhibitors (including fluoxetine and sertraline). In general, antidepressants produce fewer adverse effects than do amphetamines. But troublesome side effects still occur in some patients, including impotence, high blood pressure, and heart rhythm irregularities.

On July 17, 2002, the FDA approved Xyrem (sodium oxybate or gamma hydroxybutyrate, also known as GHB) for treating people with narcolepsy who experience episodes of cataplexy. Due to safety concerns associated with the use of this drug, the distribution of Xyrem is tightly restricted.

What behavioral strategies help people cope with symptoms?

None of the currently available medications enables people with narcolepsy to consistently maintain a fully normal state of alertness. Thus, drug therapy should be supplemented by various behavioral strategies according to the needs of the individual patient.

> ### ♣ It's A Fact!!
>
> People with narcolepsy can work in almost all types of jobs. It may be best if you have a flexible work schedule so you can take naps when needed. It also helps to have a job where you interact with your coworkers. Try to avoid jobs that require you to drive or have long commutes to work.
>
> Source: Excerpted from "Narcolepsy," National Heart, Lung, and Blood Institute, 2006.

To gain greater control over their symptoms, many patients take short, regularly scheduled naps at times when they tend to feel sleepiest. Adults can often negotiate with employers to modify their work schedules so they can take naps when necessary and perform their most demanding tasks when they are most alert. The Americans with Disabilities Act requires employers to provide reasonable accommodations for all employees with disabilities. Children and adolescents with narcolepsy can be similarly accommodated through modifying class schedules and informing school personnel of special needs, including medication requirements during the school day.

Improving the quality of nighttime sleep can combat EDS and help relieve persistent feelings of fatigue. Among the most important common-sense measures patients can take to enhance sleep quality are: maintaining a regular sleep schedule; avoiding alcohol and caffeine-containing beverages for several hours before bedtime; avoiding smoking, especially at night; maintaining a comfortable, adequately warmed bedroom environment; and engaging in relaxing activities such as a warm bath before bedtime. Exercising for at least 20 minutes per day at least four or five hours before bedtime also improves sleep quality and can help people with narcolepsy avoid gaining excess weight.

Safety precautions, particularly when driving, are of paramount importance for all persons with narcolepsy. Although the disorder, in itself, is not fatal, EDS and cataplexy can lead to serious injury or death if left uncontrolled. Suddenly falling asleep or losing muscle control can transform actions that are ordinarily safe, such as walking down a long flight of stairs, into hazards. People with untreated narcoleptic symptoms are involved in automobile accidents roughly 10 times more frequently than the general population. However, accident rates are normal among patients who have received appropriate medication.

Finally, patient support groups frequently prove extremely beneficial because people with narcolepsy may become socially isolated due to embarrassment about their symptoms. Many patients also attempt to avoid experiencing strong emotions, since humor, excitement, and other intense feelings can trigger cataplectic attacks. Moreover, because of the widespread lack of public knowledge about the disorder, people with narcolepsy are too often unfairly judged to be lazy, unintelligent, undisciplined, or unmotivated. Such stigmatization often increases the tendency toward self-imposed isolation. The empathy and understanding that support groups offer people can be crucial to their overall sense of well-being and provide them with a network of social contacts who can offer practical help and emotional support.

♣ It's A Fact!!
School-Aged Children

Narcolepsy symptoms can affect learning by limiting children's ability to study, focus, and remember. Children with narcolepsy are sometimes mistakenly thought to have a learning disability or a seizure disorder (epilepsy). When tired, some children with narcolepsy tend to speed up their activities, rather than slow down. These children can be mistakenly labeled as hyperactive.

You might want to tell your teachers and school administrators about the narcolepsy. It is also helpful to tell the school nurse about the condition and the medicines you take for it. Together you can work out a place to keep the medicines and a schedule for taking them at school. You also might want to check with student services about special education and other services, if needed.

Source: Excerpted from "Narcolepsy," National Heart, Lung, and Blood Institute, 2006.

✔ Quick Tip

Driving can be dangerous for people with narcolepsy. You need to take special care to help prevent crashes:

- Take medicines as prescribed.

- Ask your doctor if you can drive safely.

- Plan to drive when you are least likely to have a sleep attack or other narcolepsy symptom that could be dangerous while driving.

- Take naps before driving.

- Stop regularly during a long drive and exercise during the stops.

- Consider driving with family, friends, or coworkers or getting rides from them.

Source: Excerpted from "Narcolepsy," National Heart, Lung, and Blood Institute, 2006.

What research is being done?

Within the Federal government, the National Institute of Neurological Disorders and Stroke (NINDS), a component of the National Institutes of Health (NIH), has primary responsibility for sponsoring research on neurological disorders. As part of its mission, the NINDS supports research on narcolepsy and other sleep disorders with a neurological basis through grants to major medical institutions across the country.

Within the National Heart, Lung, and Blood Institute, also a component of the NIH, the National Center on Sleep Disorders Research (NCSDR) coordinates Federal government sleep research activities and shares information with private and nonprofit groups. NCSDR staff also promote doctoral and postdoctoral training programs, and educates the public and health care professional about sleep disorders. For more information, go to the NCSDR website at http://www.nhlbi.nih.gov/about/ncsdr/index.htm.

NINDS-sponsored researchers are conducting studies devoted to further clarifying the wide range of genetic factors—both HLA genes and non-HLA genes—that may cause narcolepsy. Other scientists are conducting investigations using animal models to identify neurotransmitters other than the hypocretins that may contribute to disease development. A greater understanding of the complex genetic and biochemical bases of narcolepsy will eventually lead to the formulation of new therapies to control symptoms and may lead to a cure. Researchers are also investigating the modes of action of wake-promoting compounds to widen the range of available therapeutic options.

Scientists have long suspected that abnormal immunological processes may be an important element in the cause of narcolepsy, but until recently clear evidence supporting this suspicion has been lacking. NINDS-sponsored scientists have recently uncovered evidence demonstrating the presence of unusual, possibly pathological, forms of immunological activity in narcoleptic

---

🖙 Remember!!

- Narcolepsy is a lifelong condition that causes you to fall asleep suddenly during the day.

- Narcolepsy may cause sudden loss of muscle tone and control while awake (cataplexy), the inability to move or speak while falling asleep or waking up (sleep paralysis), and/or vivid dreams while falling asleep or waking up (hallucinations).

- The symptoms of narcolepsy can cause accidents; injuries; and problems with learning, working, or connecting with others.

- Narcolepsy tends to develop first between the ages of 15 and 30.

- The exact causes of narcolepsy are not known. Many factors probably work together to cause a lack of the brain chemical hypocretin, which promotes wakefulness.

- A diagnosis of narcolepsy is based on symptoms, family history of narcolepsy, and the results of sleep tests.

- There is no cure for narcolepsy, but its symptoms can be relieved with medicines and lifestyle changes.

- Most people with narcolepsy can lead near-normal lives.

- People with narcolepsy have a number of sources of support. These include laws that may provide them more flexibility at work and financial or insurance support, if needed. There are also patient support groups, such as the Narcolepsy Network (http://www.narcolepsynetwork.org).

Source: Excerpted from "Narcolepsy," National Heart, Lung, and Blood Institute, 2006.

dogs. These researchers are now investigating whether drugs that suppress immunological processes may interrupt the development of narcolepsy in this animal model.

Recently there has been a growing awareness that narcolepsy can develop during childhood and may contribute to the development of behavior disorders. A group of NINDS-sponsored scientists is now conducting a large epidemiological study to determine the prevalence of narcolepsy in children aged two to fourteen years who have been diagnosed with attention deficit hyperactivity disorder.

Finally, the NINDS continues to support investigations into the basic biology of sleep, including the brain mechanisms involved in generating and regulating REM sleep. Scientists are now examining physiological processes occurring in a portion of the hindbrain called the amygdala in order to uncover novel biochemical processes underlying REM sleep. A more comprehensive understanding of the complex biology of sleep will undoubtedly further clarify the pathological processes that underlie narcolepsy and other sleep disorders.

Chapter 23

Hypersomnia And Kleine-Levin Syndrome

Hypersomnia

What is hypersomnia?

Hypersomnia is characterized by recurrent episodes of excessive daytime sleepiness or prolonged nighttime sleep. Different from feeling tired due to lack of or interrupted sleep at night, persons with hypersomnia are compelled to nap repeatedly during the day, often at inappropriate times such as at work, during a meal, or in conversation. These daytime naps usually provide no relief from symptoms. Patients often have difficulty waking from a long sleep, and may feel disoriented. Other symptoms may include anxiety, increased irritation, decreased energy, restlessness, slow thinking, slow speech, loss of appetite, hallucinations, and memory difficulty. Some patients lose the ability to function in family, social, occupational, or other settings. Hypersomnia may be caused by another sleep disorder (such as narcolepsy or sleep apnea), dysfunction of the autonomic nervous system, or drug or alcohol abuse. In some cases it results from a physical problem, such as a tumor, head trauma, or injury to the central nervous system. Certain medications, or medicine withdrawal, may also cause hypersomnia. Medical conditions including multiple sclerosis, depression, encephalitis, epilepsy, or obesity may

About This Chapter: Both of the following documents are provided by the National Institute of Neurological Disorders and Stroke (NINDS), February 13, 2007: "NINDS Hypersomnia Information Page" and "NINDS Kleine-Levin Syndrome Information Page."

contribute to the disorder. Some people appear to have a genetic predisposition to hypersomnia; in others, there is no known cause. Hypersomnia typically affects adolescents and young adults.

Is there any treatment?

Treatment is symptomatic in nature. Stimulants, such as amphetamine, methylphenidate, and modafinil, may be prescribed. Other drugs used to treat hypersomnia include clonidine, levodopa, bromocriptine, antidepressants, and monoamine oxidase inhibitors. Changes in behavior (for example avoiding night work and social activities that delay bed time) and diet may offer some relief. Patients should avoid alcohol and caffeine.

What is the prognosis?

The prognosis for persons with hypersomnia depends on the cause of the disorder. While the disorder itself is not life threatening, it can have serious consequences, such as automobile accidents caused by falling asleep while driving. The attacks usually continue indefinitely.

What research is being done?

The National Institute of Neurological Disorders and Stroke (NINDS) supports and conducts research on sleep disorders such as hypersomnia. The goal of this research is to increase scientific understanding of the condition, find improved methods of diagnosing and treating it, and discover ways to prevent it.

Kleine-Levin Syndrome

What is Kleine-Levin syndrome?

Kleine-Levin syndrome is a rare disorder that causes recurring periods of excessive drowsiness and sleep (up to 20 hours per day). Symptoms, which may last for days to weeks, include excessive food intake, irritability, disorientation, lack of energy, and hypersensitivity to noise. Some patients may also experience hallucinations and an abnormally uninhibited sex drive. Affected persons are normal between episodes, although depression and amnesia may be noted temporarily after an attack. It may be weeks or more before symptoms reappear. Onset is typically around adolescence to the late teens.

Symptoms may be related to malfunction of the hypothalamus, the part of the brain that governs appetite and sleep.

Is there any treatment?

There is no definitive treatment for Kleine-Levin syndrome. Stimulants, including amphetamines, methylphenidate, and modafinil, administered orally, are used to treat sleepiness. Because of similarities between Kleine-Levin syndrome and certain mood disorders, lithium and carbamazepine may be prescribed. Responses to treatment have often been limited. This disorder needs to be differentiated from cyclic re-occurrence of sleepiness during the premenstrual period in teenaged girls that may be controlled with birth control pills.

♣ **It's A Fact!!**

Kleine-Levin syndrome is four times more common in males than in females.

Source: "NINDS Kleine-Levin Syndrome Information Page," National Institute of Neurological Disorders and Stroke, February 13, 2007.

What is the prognosis?

The disorder appears to be benign and does not impact on intellect or physical function. Symptoms usually improve or disappear with advancing age.

What research is being done?

NINDS supports a broad range of clinical and basic research on diseases causing sleep disorders, in an effort to clarify the mechanisms of these conditions and to develop better treatments for them.

Chapter 24

Restless Legs Syndrome

What is restless legs?

Restless legs syndrome (RLS) is a neurological disorder characterized by unpleasant sensations in the legs and an uncontrollable urge to move when at rest in an effort to relieve these feelings. RLS sensations are often described by people as burning, creeping, tugging, or like insects crawling inside the legs. Often called paresthesias (abnormal sensations) or dysesthesias (unpleasant abnormal sensations), the sensations range in severity from uncomfortable to irritating to painful.

The most distinctive or unusual aspect of the condition is that lying down and trying to relax activates the symptoms. As a result, most people with RLS have difficulty falling asleep and staying asleep. Left untreated, the condition causes exhaustion and daytime fatigue. Many people with RLS report that their job, personal relations, and activities of daily living are strongly affected as a result of their exhaustion. They are often unable to concentrate, have impaired memory, or fail to accomplish daily tasks.

Some researchers estimate that RLS affects as many as 12 million Americans. However, others estimate a much higher occurrence because RLS is thought to be under-diagnosed and, in some cases, misdiagnosed.

About This Chapter: "Restless Legs Syndrome Fact Sheet," National Institute of Neurological Disorders and Stroke, February 14, 2007.

Some people with RLS will not seek medical attention, believing that they will not be taken seriously, that their symptoms are too mild, or that their condition is not treatable. Some physicians wrongly attribute the symptoms to nervousness, insomnia, stress, arthritis, muscle cramps, or aging.

RLS occurs in both genders, although the incidence may be slightly higher in women. Although the syndrome may begin at any age, even as early as infancy, most patients who are severely affected are middle-aged or older. In addition, the severity of the disorder appears to increase with age. Older patients experience symptoms more frequently and for longer periods of time.

More than 80 percent of people with RLS also experience a more common condition known as periodic limb movement disorder (PLMD). PLMD is characterized by involuntary leg twitching or jerking movements during sleep that typically occur every 10 to 60 seconds, sometimes throughout the night. The symptoms cause repeated awakening and severely disrupted sleep. Unlike RLS, the movements caused by PLMD are involuntary—people have no control over them. Although many patients with RLS also develop PLMD, most people with PLMD do not experience RLS. Like RLS, the cause of PLMD is unknown.

✤ It's A Fact!!

There are two types of RLS:

- Primary RLS is the most common type of RLS. It is also called idiopathic RLS. "Primary" means the cause is not known. Primary RLS, once it starts, usually becomes a lifelong condition. Over time, symptoms tend to get worse and occur more often, especially if they began in childhood or early in adult life. In milder cases, there may be long periods of time with no symptoms, or symptoms may last only for a limited time.

- Secondary RLS is RLS that is caused by another disease or condition or, sometimes, from taking certain medicines. Symptoms usually go away when the disease or condition improves, or if the medicine is stopped.

Source: "Restless Leg Syndrome," National Institute of Heart, Lung, and Blood Institute, 2005.

What are common signs and symptoms of restless legs?

As described previously, people with RLS feel uncomfortable sensations in their legs, especially when sitting or lying down, accompanied by an irresistible urge to move about. These sensations usually occur deep inside the leg, between the knee and ankle; more rarely, they occur in the feet, thighs, arms, and hands. Although the sensations can occur on just one side of the body, they most often affect both sides.

Because moving the legs (or other affected parts of the body) relieves the discomfort, people with RLS often keep their legs in motion to minimize or prevent the sensations. They may pace the floor, constantly move their legs while sitting, and toss and turn in bed.

Most people find the symptoms to be less noticeable during the day and more pronounced in the evening or at night, especially during the onset of sleep. For many people, the symptoms disappear by early morning, allowing for more refreshing sleep at that time. Other triggering situations are periods of inactivity such as long car trips, sitting in a movie theater, long-distance flights, immobilization in a cast, or relaxation exercises.

The symptoms of RLS vary in severity and duration from person to person. Mild RLS occurs episodically, with only mild disruption of sleep onset, and causes little distress. In moderately severe cases, symptoms occur only once or twice a week but result in significant delay of sleep onset, with some disruption of daytime function. In severe cases of RLS, the symptoms occur more than twice a week and result in burdensome interruption of sleep and impairment of daytime function.

Symptoms may begin at any stage of life, although the disorder is more common with increasing age. Sometimes people will experience spontaneous improvement over a period of weeks or months. Although rare, spontaneous improvement over a period of years also can occur. If these improvements occur, it is usually during the early stages of the disorder. In general, however, symptoms become more severe over time.

People who have both RLS and an associated condition tend to develop more severe symptoms rapidly. In contrast, those whose RLS is not related to any other medical condition and whose onset is at an early age show a very slow progression of the disorder and many years may pass before symptoms occur regularly.

What causes restless legs syndrome?

In most cases, the cause of RLS is unknown (referred to as idiopathic). A family history of the condition is seen in approximately 50 percent of such cases, suggesting a genetic form of the disorder. People with familial RLS tend to be younger when symptoms start and have a slower progression of the condition.

In other cases, RLS appears to be related to the following factors or conditions, although researchers do not yet know if these factors actually cause RLS.

• People with low iron levels or anemia may be prone to developing RLS. Once iron levels or anemia is corrected, patients may see a reduction in symptoms.

• Chronic diseases such as kidney failure, diabetes, Parkinson disease, and peripheral neuropathy are associated with RLS. Treating the underlying condition often provides relief from RLS symptoms.

• Some pregnant women experience RLS, especially in their last trimester. For most of these women, symptoms usually disappear within four weeks after delivery.

♣ It's A Fact!!
Periodic Limb Movement Disorder

Most people with RLS also have a condition called periodic limb movement disorder (PLMD). PLMD is a condition in which a person's legs twitch or jerk uncontrollably about every 10 to 60 seconds. This usually happens during sleep. These movements cause repeated awakenings that disturb or reduce sleep. PLMD usually affects the legs but can also affect the arms.

Source: "Restless Leg Syndrome," National Institute of Heart, Lung, and Blood Institute, 2005.

- Certain medications—such as antinausea drugs (prochlorperazine or metoclopramide), anti-seizure drugs (phenytoin or droperidol), antipsychotic drugs (haloperidol or phenothiazine derivatives), and some cold and allergy medications—may aggravate symptoms. Patients can talk with their physicians about the possibility of changing medications.

Researchers also have found that caffeine, alcohol, and tobacco may aggravate or trigger symptoms in patients who are predisposed to develop RLS. Some studies have shown that a reduction or complete elimination of such substances may relieve symptoms, although it remains unclear whether elimination of such substances can prevent RLS symptoms from occurring at all.

How is restless legs syndrome diagnosed?

Currently, there is no single diagnostic test for RLS. The disorder is diagnosed clinically by evaluating the patient's history and symptoms. Despite a clear description of clinical features, the condition is often misdiagnosed or under-diagnosed. In 1995, the International Restless Legs Syndrome Study Group identified four basic criteria for diagnosing RLS: (1) a desire to move the limbs, often associated with paresthesias or dysesthesias, (2) symptoms that are worse or present only during rest and are partially or temporarily relieved by activity, (3) motor restlessness, and (4) nocturnal worsening of symptoms. Although about 80 percent of those with RLS also experience PLMD, it is not necessary for a diagnosis of RLS. In more severe cases, patients may experience dyskinesia (uncontrolled, often continuous movements) while awake, and some experience symptoms in one or both of their arms as well as their legs. Most people with RLS have sleep disturbances, largely because of the limb discomfort and jerking. The result is excessive daytime sleepiness and fatigue.

Despite these efforts to establish standard criteria, the clinical diagnosis of RLS is difficult to make. Physicians must rely largely on patients' descriptions of symptoms and information from their medical history, including past medical problems, family history, and current medications. Patients may be asked about frequency, duration, and intensity of symptoms as well as their tendency toward daytime sleep patterns and sleepiness, disturbance of sleep, or daytime function. If a patient's history is suggestive of RLS, laboratory tests may be performed to rule out other conditions and support the diagnosis of RLS. Blood tests to exclude anemia, decreased iron stores, diabetes, and renal dysfunction should be performed. Electromyography and nerve conduction studies may also be recommended to measure electrical activity in muscles and nerves, and Doppler sonography may be used to evaluate muscle activity in the legs. Such tests can document any accompanying damage or disease in nerves and nerve roots (such as peripheral neuropathy and radiculopathy) or other leg-related movement disorders. Negative results from tests may indicate that the diagnosis is RLS. In some cases, sleep studies such as polysomnography are undertaken to identify the presence of PLMD.

✎ What's It Mean?

Polysomnography: A test that records the patient's brain waves, heartbeat, and breathing during an entire night.

Source: National Institute of Neurological Disorders and Stroke, February 14, 2007.

The diagnosis is especially difficult with children because the physician relies heavily on the patient's explanations of symptoms, which, given the nature of the symptoms of RLS, can be difficult for a child to describe. The syndrome can sometimes be misdiagnosed as "growing pains" or attention deficit disorder.

How is restless legs syndrome treated?

Although movement brings relief to those with RLS, it is generally only temporary. However, RLS can be controlled by finding any possible underlying disorder. Often, treating the associated medical condition, such as peripheral neuropathy or diabetes, will alleviate many symptoms. For patients with idiopathic RLS, treatment is directed toward relieving symptoms.

For those with mild to moderate symptoms, prevention is key, and many physicians suggest certain lifestyle changes and activities to reduce or eliminate symptoms. Decreased use of caffeine, alcohol, and tobacco may provide some relief. Physicians may suggest that certain individuals take supplements to correct deficiencies in iron, folate, and magnesium. Studies also have shown that maintaining a regular sleep pattern can reduce symptoms. Some individuals, finding that RLS symptoms are minimized in the early morning, change their sleep patterns. Others have found that a program of regular moderate exercise helps them sleep better; on the other hand, excessive exercise has been reported by some patients to aggravate RLS symptoms. Taking a hot bath, massaging the legs, or using a heating pad or ice pack can help relieve symptoms in some patients. Although many patients find some relief with such measures, rarely do these efforts completely eliminate symptoms.

Physicians also may suggest a variety of medications to treat RLS. Generally, physicians choose from dopaminergics, benzodiazepines (central nervous system depressants), opioids, and anticonvulsants. Dopaminergic agents, largely used to treat Parkinson disease, have been shown to reduce RLS symptoms and PLMD and are considered the initial treatment of choice. Good short-term results of treatment with levodopa plus carbidopa have been reported, although most patients eventually will develop augmentation, meaning that symptoms are reduced at night but begin to develop earlier in the day than usual. Dopamine agonists such as pergolide mesylate, pramipexole, and ropinirole hydrochloride may be effective in some patients and are less likely to cause augmentation.

In 2005, ropinirole became the only drug approved by the U.S. Food and Drug Administration specifically for the treatment of moderate to severe RLS. The drug was first approved in 1997 for patients with Parkinson disease.

Benzodiazepines (such as clonazepam and diazepam) may be prescribed for patients who have mild or intermittent symptoms. These drugs help patients obtain a more restful sleep but they do not fully alleviate RLS symptoms and can cause daytime sleepiness. Because these depressants also may induce or aggravate sleep apnea in some cases, they should not be used in people with this condition.

For more severe symptoms, opioids such as codeine, propoxyphene, or oxycodone may be prescribed for their ability to induce relaxation and diminish pain. Side effects include dizziness, nausea, vomiting, and the risk of addiction.

Anticonvulsants such as carbamazepine and gabapentin are also useful for some patients, as they decrease the sensory disturbances (creeping and crawling sensations). Dizziness, fatigue, and sleepiness are among the possible side effects.

Unfortunately, no one drug is effective for everyone with RLS. What may be helpful to one individual may actually worsen symptoms for another. In addition, medications taken regularly may lose their effect, making it necessary to change medications periodically.

What is the prognosis of people with restless legs?

RLS is generally a lifelong condition for which there is no cure. Symptoms may gradually worsen with age, though more slowly for those with the idiopathic form of RLS than for patients who also suffer from an associated medical condition. Nevertheless, current therapies can control the disorder, minimizing symptoms and increasing periods of restful sleep. In addition, some patients have remissions, periods in which symptoms decrease or disappear for days, weeks, or months, although symptoms usually eventually reappear. A diagnosis of RLS does not indicate the onset of another neurological disease.

What research is being done?

Within the Federal Government, the National Institute of Neurological Disorders and Stroke (NINDS), one of the National Institutes of Health,

♣ It's A Fact!! Living With Restless Legs Syndrome

Restless legs syndrome (RLS) is often a lifelong condition. The symptoms may come and go frequently or disappear completely for long periods of time. They may get worse over time. Lifestyle changes and medicines can help control and relieve the symptoms of RLS. For severe symptoms, ongoing medicines may be needed. Talk with your doctor about lifestyle changes and medicines that might help your symptoms. New treatments are being developed as research continues.

Source: "Restless Leg Syndrome," National Institute of Heart, Lung, and Blood Institute, 2005.

has primary responsibility for conducting and supporting research on RLS. The goal of this research is to increase scientific understanding of RLS, find improved methods of diagnosing and treating the syndrome, and discover ways to prevent it.

NINDS-supported researchers are investigating the possible role of dopamine function in RLS. Dopamine is a chemical messenger responsible for transmitting signals between one area of the brain, the substantia nigra, and the next relay station of the brain, the corpus striatum, to produce smooth, purposeful muscle activity. Researchers suspect that impaired transmission of dopamine signals may play a role in RLS. Additional research should provide new information about how RLS occurs and may help investigators identify more successful treatment options.

The NINDS sponsored a workshop on dopamine in 1999 to help plan a course for future research on disorders such as RLS and recommend ways to advance and encourage research in this field. Participants' recommendations for further research included the development of an animal model of RLS; additional genetic, epidemiologic, and pathophysiologic investigations of RLS; efforts to define genetic and non-genetic forms of RLS; establishment of a brain tissue bank to aid investigators; continuing investigations on dopamine and RLS; and studies of PLMD as it relates to RLS.

Research on pallidotomy, a surgical procedure in which a portion of the brain called the globus pallidus is lesioned, may contribute to a greater understanding of the pathophysiology of RLS and may lead to a possible treatment. A recent study by NINDS-funded researchers showed that a patient with RLS and Parkinson disease benefited from a pallidotomy and obtained relief from the limb discomfort caused by RLS. Additional research must be conducted to duplicate these results in other patients and to learn whether pallidotomy would be effective in RLS patients who do not also have Parkinson disease.

In other related research, NINDS scientists are conducting studies with patients to better understand the physiological mechanisms of PLMD associated with RLS.

☞ Remember!!

- Restless legs syndrome (RLS) is a sensory disorder causing an almost irresistible urge to move the legs. The urge to move the legs is usually due to unpleasant feelings in the legs that occur when at rest. Movement eases the feelings but only for a while.

- Symptoms of RLS can range from mild to severe. Symptoms tend to get worse over time. They sometimes begin during childhood.

- People with RLS may describe the unpleasant feelings in their legs as creeping, crawling, tingling, burning, or painful. Often, the feelings are hard to describe.

- Many people with RLS also have periodic limb movement disorder. This is a condition in which a person's legs twitch or jerk uncontrollably every 10 to 60 seconds. This usually happens during sleep.

- RLS can make it difficult to fall asleep and stay asleep. People with RLS often don't get enough sleep and may feel tired and sleepy during the day.

- There are two types of RLS: primary and secondary.

- In primary RLS the cause is not known. However, it tends to run in families.

- Secondary RLS is RLS that is caused by another disease or condition or, sometimes, by taking certain medicines.

- RLS is common in pregnant women. It usually occurs during the last 3 months of pregnancy and usually improves or disappears within a few weeks after delivery.

- Lifestyle changes can improve and relieve symptoms of RLS. Lifestyle changes may be the only treatment needed for mild symptoms of RLS.

- Medicines can help to treat more severe symptoms of RLS. No single medicine is helpful in all persons with RLS. It may take several changes in medicines and dosages to find the best approach.

Source: "Restless Leg Syndrome," National Institute of Heart, Lung, and Blood Institute, 2005.

Chapter 25

Sleepwalking

Eleven-year-old Cait was trying to fall asleep when her 8-year-old brother, Doug, came into her room. He said, "Cait, I'll babysit all your dolls. I'll take good care of them. You have to give them to me."

She didn't understand what he meant and when she asked, "What do you mean?" he mumbled something that sounded like "caterpillar." Then Doug went back into the hallway and stood there staring up at the hall light.

Little brothers can be weird, but this was really strange. Cait didn't know what to do. Just then, Cait's father appeared and explained that Doug was sleepwalking.

What is sleepwalking?

Not all sleep is the same every night. We experience some deep, quiet sleep and some active sleep, which is when dreams happen. You might think sleepwalking would happen during active sleep, but a person isn't physically active during active sleep. Sleepwalking usually happens in the first few hours of sleep in the stage called slow-wave or deep sleep.

About This Chapter: This information was provided by TeensHealth, one of the largest resources online for medically reviewed health information written for parents, kids, and teens. For more articles like this one, visit www.TeensHealth.org, or www.KidsHealth.org. © 2004 The Nemours Foundation.

Not all sleepwalkers actually walk. Some simply sit up or stand in bed or act like they're awake (but dazed) when in fact, they're asleep! Most, however, do get up and move around for a few seconds or for as long as half an hour.

Sleepwalkers' eyes are open, but they don't see the same way they do when they're awake and often think they're in different rooms of the house or different places altogether. Sleepwalkers tend to go back to bed on their own and they won't remember it in the morning.

♣ **It's A Fact!!**
Researchers estimate that about 15% of kids sleepwalk regularly. Sleepwalking may run in families and sometimes occurs when a person is sick, has a fever, is not getting enough sleep, or is stressed.

Is sleepwalking a serious problem?

If sleepwalking occurs frequently, every night or so, it's a good idea for your mom or dad to take you to see your doctor. But occasional sleepwalking generally isn't something to worry about, although it may look funny or even scary for the people who see a sleepwalker in action.

Although occasional sleepwalking isn't a big deal, it's important, of course, that the person is kept safe. Precautions should be taken so the person is less likely to fall down, run into something, or walk out the front door while sleepwalking.

What will the doctor do?

There's no cure for sleepwalking, but the doctor can talk to you about what's happening and try to find ways to help you sleep more soundly. Most children just grow out of sleepwalking.

For kids who sleepwalk often, doctors may recommend a treatment called scheduled awakening. This disrupts the sleep cycle enough to help stop sleepwalking. In rare cases, a doctor may prescribe medication to help the person sleep.

Here are some tips to help prevent sleepwalking:

• Relax at bedtime by listening to soft music or relaxation tapes.

- Have a regular sleep schedule and stick to it.

- Keep noise to a minimum while you're trying to sleep.

- Avoid drinking a lot in the evening and be sure to go to the bathroom before going to bed. (A full bladder can contribute to sleepwalking.)

How do I take care of a sleepwalker?

One thing you can do to help a sleepwalker is to clear rooms and hallways of furniture or obstacles they might encounter if they sleepwalk during the night. If there are stairs or dangerous areas, a grown-up should close doors and windows or install safety gates.

You also may have heard that sleepwalkers can get really scared if you startle them into being awake. That's true, so what do you do if you see someone sleepwalking? You should call for a grown-up who can gently steer the person back to bed. And once the sleepwalking person is tucked back in bed, it's time for you to get some shut-eye, too.

Chapter 26

Nocturnal Sleep-Related Eating Disorder

There are at least two problems that involve disordered eating primarily at night: nocturnal sleep-related eating disorder, which is discussed here, and night eating syndrome, which is described later in this chapter. The Anorexia Nervosa and Related Eating Disorders, Inc. (ANRED) suggests you read the material on both so you will have a better understanding of these perplexing and distressing problems.

When I woke up this morning, there were candy bar wrappers all over the kitchen, and I had a stomach ache. I had chocolate on my face and hands. My husband says I was up eating last night, but I have no memories of doing so. Could he be playing a joke on me?

Maybe not. You might have nocturnal sleep-related eating disorder, a relatively unknown condition currently being investigated.

What is nocturnal sleep-related eating disorder (NS-RED)?

In spite of its name, NS-RED is not, strictly speaking, an eating disorder. It is thought to be a type of sleep disorder in which people eat while seeming to be sound asleep. They may eat in bed or roam through the house and prowl the kitchen.

About This Chapter: This chapter includes "Nocturnal Sleep-Related Eating Disorder" and "Night Eating Syndrome," used with permission of ANRED: Anorexia Nervosa and Related Eating Disorders, Inc., http://www.anred.com, © 2006.

These people are not conscious during episodes of NS-RED, which may be related to sleep-walking. They are not aware that they are eating. They have no memories of having done so when they wake, or they have only fragmentary memories. Episodes seem to occur in a state somewhere between wakefulness and sleep.

When people with NS-RED awake and discover the evidence of their nighttime forays, they are embarrassed, ashamed, and afraid they may be losing their minds. Some, when confronted with the evidence by family members, deny that they were the perpetrators. They truly do not believe they could have done such a thing and cannot admit to such dramatic loss of control.

> ♣ **It's A Fact!!**
>
> Sleep disorders, including NS-RED, seem to run in families. They may have a genetic component.
>
> Source: "Nocturnal Sleep-Related Eating Disorder," © 2006 ANRED: Anorexia Nervosa and Related Eating Disorders, Inc.

Food consumed during NS-RED episodes tends to be high-fat, high-sugar comfort food that people deny themselves while awake. Sometimes these folks eat bizarre combinations of food (hotdogs dipped in peanut butter, raw bacon smeared with mayonnaise, etc.) or non-food items like soap that they have sliced like they would slice cheese.

Who gets NS-RED?

One to three percent of the general population (3 to 9 million people) seems to be subject to this disorder, and ten to fifteen percent of people with eating disorders are affected. The problem may be chronic or appear once or twice and then disappear. Many of these people are severely stressed, anxious individuals who are dismayed and angry at themselves for their nocturnal loss of control. Their behaviors may pave the way to depression and weight gain.

Many of these individuals diet during the day, which leaves them hungry and vulnerable to binge eating at night when their control is weakened by sleep.

People with NS-RED sometimes have histories of alcoholism, drug abuse, and sleep disorders other than NS-RED, problems such as sleep walking, restless legs, and sleep apnea. Their sleep is fragmented, and they are often tired when they wake.

Reports have been received by the FDA and the makers of Ambien, a prescription sleep aid, to the effect that some of the people who took this medication discovered that they had eaten or binge eaten while they slept under the influence of the drug. Most had no memory of doing so when they awoke in the morning. A scientific paper is pending. For more information see *Newsweek*, March 27, 2006, p.54.

How can people eat and not remember doing so? Are they lying?

No, they are not lying. It seems that parts of their brains are truly asleep, and, at the same time, other parts are awake. The parts that regulate waking consciousness are asleep, so the next day there are no memories of eating the night before.

Is there any treatment for NS-RED? If there is, what is it?

Yes, there is treatment. It begins with a clinical interview and a night or two at a sleep-disorders center where brain activity is monitored. Sometimes medication is helpful, but sleeping pills should be avoided. They can make matters worse by increasing confusion and clumsiness that can lead to injury. Regular use of sleeping pills can also lead to dependency and rebound wakefulness on withdrawal. Instead, ask your doctor about prescription selective serotonin reuptake inhibitors (SSRIs).

Also helpful are interventions that reduce stress and anxiety; for example, stress management classes, assertiveness training, counseling, and reducing intake of alcohol, street drugs, and caffeine.

How about self-help techniques? Are there any that work?

Some people find that sleep-eating episodes are fewer and farther between if they play soft, rhythmic music at night. Headsets and earbuds can eliminate annoyance for bed partners, but the volume should be low enough to prevent damage to one's hearing.

Some people enlist the help of family members who lock cupboards and the refrigerator at night and then hide the keys. Others tie one end of a thread or string to a wrist and the other to the bed frame so that they wake themselves if they get up and walk away from the bed. Some have even used baby alarms or burglar alarms that are triggered by motion.

These techniques should be implemented carefully and safely so that a person who is somewhere between sleep and wakefulness does not hurt her/himself during a sleep-walking/eating episode.

✔ **Quick Tip**

If you think you may have NS-RED, before you try self-help, talk to your physician and ask for a referral to a sleep-disorders treatment center. You especially need to talk to your doctor if you are taking, or have taken, the sleep medication Ambien. Help is available. Take advantage of it.

Source: "Nocturnal Sleep-Related Eating Disorder," © 2006 ANRED: Anorexia Nervosa and Related Eating Disorders, Inc.

Night Eating Syndrome

There are at least two problems that involve disordered eating primarily at night: night eating syndrome, which is discussed here, and nocturnal sleep-related eating disorder, which is described above. The Anorexia Nervosa and Related Eating Disorders, Inc. (ANRED) suggests you read the material on both so you will have a better understanding of these perplexing and distressing problems.

Signs And Symptoms

• The person has little or no appetite for breakfast. Delays first meal for several hours after waking up. Is not hungry or is upset about how much was eaten the night before.

• Eats more food after dinner than during that meal.

- Eats more than half of daily food intake during and after dinner but before breakfast. May wake up and leave the bed to snack at night. May not be aware at the time of what they are doing.

- This pattern has persisted for at least two months.

- Person feels tense, anxious, upset, or guilty while eating.

- Night eating syndrome (NES) is thought to be stress related and is often accompanied by depression. Especially at night the person may be moody, tense, anxious, nervous, agitated, etc.

- Has trouble falling asleep or staying asleep. Wakes frequently and then often eats.

- Foods ingested are often carbohydrates: sugary and starchy.

- Behavior is not like binge eating which is done in relatively short episodes. Night eating syndrome involves continual eating throughout evening hours.

- This eating produces guilt and shame, not enjoyment.

Discussion

Night-eating syndrome (NES) has not yet been formally defined as an eating disorder. Underlying causes are being identified, and treatment plans are still being developed. It seems likely that a combination of biological, genetic, and emotional factors contribute to the problem.

♣ **It's A Fact!!**
How many people have night-eating syndrome?

Perhaps only one to two percent (1–2%) of adults in the general population have this problem, but research at the University of Pennsylvania School of Medicine suggests that about six percent of people who seek treatment for obesity have NES. Another study suggests that more than a quarter (27%) of people who are overweight by at least 100 pounds have the problem.

Source: "Night Eating Syndrome," © 2006 ANRED: Anorexia Nervosa and Related Eating Disorders, Inc.

One theory postulates that people with this condition are under stress, either recognized or hidden. Their bodies are flooded with cortisol, a stress hormone. Eating may be the body's attempt to neutralize cortisol or slow down its production. More research needs to be done before this explanation can be accepted or rejected. In any event, stress appears to be a cause or trigger of NES, and stress-reduction programs, including mental health therapy, seem to help.

Researchers are especially interested in the foods chosen by night eaters. The heavy preference for carbohydrates, which trigger the brain to produce so-called "feel-good" neurochemicals, suggests that night eating may be an unconscious attempt to self-medicate mood problems and relieve stress.

NES may run in families. At this time is appears to respond to treatment with the SSRI sertraline (a prescription medication). NES is remarkable for characteristic disturbances in the circadian rhythm of food intake while circadian sleep rhythms remain normal.

If you are seeking help for night-eating syndrome, you would be wise to schedule a complete physical exam with your physician and also an evaluation with a counselor experienced in the treatment of eating disorders and also sleep disorders. In addition, a dietitian can help develop meal plans that distribute intake more evenly throughout the day so that you are not so vulnerable to caloric loading in the evening.

Evaluation in a sleep laboratory could be worthwhile. Most large hospitals have such facilities. It is not yet clear whether night eating is an eating disorder or sleep disorder or both. The more information available to the person and treatment team, the greater the chances are of developing an effective treatment plan.

Recent research was summarized by Albert Stunkard, M.D., University of Pennsylvania School of Medicine, at the North American Association for the Study of Obesity 2003 annual meeting, October 13, 2003. See also the January 2004 issue of the *International Journal of Eating Disorders*.

Chapter 27

Nightmares And Night Terrors

Nightmares

What are nightmares?

Nightmares are scary dreams that can wake a child leaving him or her upset and in need of comfort. They are very common in children. It is rare to find someone who has never experienced a nightmare. After a nightmare, most children are afraid to go back to sleep and often do not want to be left alone. Very young children do not know the difference between a dream and reality, so when they wake up they may not understand the concept that they were only dreaming and it is now over. They may keep insisting that something scary is still about to occur.

What causes nightmares?

Nightmares are usually a part of normal development and are a sign of a child's developing imagination. Children are also more likely to have nightmares after a frightening experience.

There are some things that can be done to help reduce the likelihood of nightmares.

About This Chapter: Text in this chapter is reprinted with permission from "Nightmares" and "Night (Sleep) Terrors," © 2007 Kidzzzsleep (www.kidzzzsleep.org). All rights reserved.

♣ It's A Fact!!
What do children and adolescents have nightmares about?

Most young toddlers have concerns about being separated from their parents. So, they may have a nightmare about being lost or having something happen to one of their parents. Nightmares also are more likely to happen following some difficult event in the child's life. For example, if a child has just started day care or her parents have gone away overnight, she is more likely to have a nightmare.

For young children, nightmares may also be the re-living of a traumatic event, such as getting lost, getting a shot at the doctor's office, or being barked at by a big dog. By age two, nightmares begin to incorporate monsters and scary things that can hurt them.

Older children often have nightmares related to scary movies or stories or a scary daytime experience.

Avoid Scary Things Before Bedtime: Don't read scary stories or watch scary movies or television shows immediately before bedtime. Choose instead a comforting bedtime routine.

Stressors: If there is something in your life that is distressing, try to take care of it. Talk to a parent or other trusted adult for reassurance. If you suddenly experience a significant increase in nightmares, try to evaluate why. Look for recurring themes that could give you a clue as to the cause and then deal with the problem.

Get Enough Sleep: Children and adolescents are much more likely to have nightmares after not getting enough sleep. So, if you are having nightmares, make sure that you are getting enough sleep as this can help decrease the frequency and intensity of nightmares.

How can you cope with nightmares?

If you have a nightmare, there are a few things that you should do:

Seek Reassurance: Comfort is the best treatment for a nightmare. Talk to a parent, guardian, or older (but compassionate) sibling. If someone is available to stay with you for a few minutes, that can help you feel safe and secure until you are ready to fall back to sleep.

Security Object: If you are attached to a security object that can be kept in bed with you, it can be beneficial and help you feel more relaxed.

Leave A Light On: If you need a light on, put it on the dimmest setting possible so you can fall back to sleep.

Discuss It The Next Day: Talk about your nightmare and see if you can figure out if anything is bothering you. Most of the time, nightmares are isolated events with little meaning, but if you start having them on a frequent basis you will want to try and figure out what is disturbing you.

Use Of Imagination: Some children and adolescents do well with using their imaginations to get rid of nightmares. You can draw pictures of your bad dreams and throw them away or you can imagine different endings. You may even find it reassuring to hang a dream catcher hung over your bed.

Get Outside Help: If your nightmares are severe, meaning that they are interfering in your life or occurring on a very frequent basis, speak to your parents, your physician, or a mental health provider.

Night (Sleep) Terrors

Night terrors are a benign (not harmful) sleep behavior, but they may cause a lot of anxiety. Night terrors are fairly common in children. Night terrors and sleepwalking often run in families. Most children outgrow night terrors by adolescence.

Night terrors occur during the stage of sleep called slow wave or deep sleep. This sleep stage is most frequent in the early part (first third) of the night. Although a child having a night terror may appear awake, he or she is really asleep.

Night terrors in children are not a sign of psychological problems. However, there are certain things, like stress, that make it more likely for someone who is prone to night terrors to have an episode. These include the following:

- not getting enough sleep

- an irregular sleep schedule

- fever or illness

- some medications

- sleeping with a full bladder

- sleeping in a different environment

- a noisy sleeping environment

♣ **It's A Fact!!**
Children with night terrors are not aware of their behavior and will not remember the night terror the next morning.

A child having a night terror may have her eyes open, and usually appears very agitated, frightened, and even panicked, as well as confused and dazed during an episode. A child will often cry out or scream at the beginning of the night terror and may mumble or give inappropriate answers to questions. A child having a night terror is often clumsy and may flail around, push a parent away, or behave in other strange ways.

Occasionally, children with night terrors get up out of bed, and can injure themselves during an episode. The sleeping environment should be made as safe as possible to avoid accidental injury. Floors should not be cluttered, objects should not be left on the stairs, and hallways should be lit. Some parents keep their child with night terrors confined to the bedroom by securely fashioning a screen door or high gate to the child's bedroom door.

The child who is having a night terror should be gently restrained to keep her safe. Generally, nothing is gained by trying to awaken a child during a night terror and sometimes doing so can make the child more agitated.

Older children and adolescents who have night terrors often spontaneously awaken. If this happens to you and your siblings (or anyone else in your family) tease you about your experiences, ask for your parents help in explaining that such teasing is not appropriate.

Children with nightly or very frequent night terrors may benefit from a treatment called scheduled awakening. This technique involves being fully awakened 30–45 minutes before the time the night terror usually occurs. This seems to interrupt the sleep cycles and decrease the chances of having a night terror.

Relaxation techniques, including relaxation tapes at bedtime, may also help prevent night terrors.

Rarely, children with very frequent or severe night terrors may need to be treated with a brief period of bedtime medication, like Valium.

If you have any questions about night terrors, or sleep in general, please ask your parents or your doctor.

Chapter 28

Enuresis (Bedwetting)

Alex falls into an extremely deep sleep almost every night. He sleeps so deeply that you could set off a fire alarm next to his bed, and he probably wouldn't hear it. Even having to pee doesn't wake up Alex, and he sometimes wets the bed while he's asleep. Alex feels embarrassed about his problem, but he's not alone. About one out of every 100 teens wets the bed. Most of them outgrow the problem, though.

What is enuresis?

The medical name for not being able to control your pee is enuresis (pronounced: en-yuh-**ree**-sis). Sometimes enuresis is also called involuntary urination. Nocturnal enuresis is involuntary urination that occurs at night. (Involuntary urination that happens during the day is known as diurnal enuresis.)

There are two kinds of enuresis: primary and secondary. If a person has primary nocturnal enuresis, that person has wet the bed since he or she was a baby. If it's secondary enuresis, the condition developed at least six months—and even several years—after a person learned to control his or her bladder.

About This Chapter: This information, from "Bedwetting (Nocturnal Enuresis)," was provided by TeensHealth, one of the largest resources online for medically reviewed health information written for parents, kids, and teens. For more articles like this one, visit www.TeensHealth.org, or www.KidsHealth.org. © 2004 The Nemours Foundation.

What causes enuresis?

The bladder is a muscular receptacle, or holding container, for pee (or urine). It expands (gets bigger) as urine enters and then contracts (gets smaller) to push the urine out.

In a person with normal bladder control, nerves in the bladder wall send a message to the brain when the bladder is full; the brain then sends a message back to the bladder to keep it from automatically emptying until the person is ready to go to the bathroom. But people with nocturnal enuresis have a problem that causes them to pee involuntarily at night.

Doctors don't always know the exact cause of nocturnal enuresis. They do have some theories, though, on what may contribute to a person developing the condition:

- **Hormonal Problems:** A hormone called antidiuretic hormone, or ADH, causes a person's body to produce less urine at night. But some people's bodies don't make enough ADH, which means their bodies may produce too much urine while they're sleeping.

- **Bladder Problems:** In some people with enuresis, too many muscle spasms can prevent the bladder from holding a normal amount of urine. Some teens and adults also have relatively small bladders that can't hold a large volume of urine.

- **Genetics:** Teens with enuresis often have a parent who had the same problem at about the same age. Scientists have identified specific genes that cause enuresis.

- **Sleep Problems.** Some teens, like Alex, may sleep so deeply that they do not wake up when they need to pee.

- **Medical Conditions:** Medical conditions that can trigger secondary enuresis include diabetes, constipation, and urinary tract infections. Spinal cord trauma, such as severe stretching of the spinal cord resulting from a fall, sports injury, auto accident, or other event may also play a role in enuresis, although this is rare. And abnormal development of the spinal cord can also lead to enuresis.

> ### ♣ It's A Fact!!
>
> Doctors don't know exactly why, but more than twice as many guys as girls have enuresis. It is frequently seen in combination with attention deficit hyperactivity disorder (ADHD).

- **Psychological Problems:** Things such as divorce, the death of a friend or family member, a move to a new town and adapting to a new school and social environment, or family tension can all feel overwhelming. It's not uncommon for people to feel stressed out during their teenage years, and stress can disturb sleep patterns.

How is enuresis diagnosed?

If you're having trouble controlling your urine at night, it's a good idea to visit the doctor to learn more about nocturnal enuresis and to rule out the possibility of a medical problem.

In addition to doing a physical examination, the doctor will ask you about any concerns and symptoms you have, your past health, your family's health, any medications you're taking, any allergies you may have, and other issues. This is called the medical history. He or she may ask about sleep patterns, bowel habits, and urinary symptoms—such as an urge to pee a lot or pain or burning when you pee. Your doctor may also discuss any stressful situations that could be contributing to the problem. If the cause appears to be emotional, the doctor may recommend that you talk with a therapist or counselor who can help get to the root of the problem.

The initial exam will probably include a screening urinalysis and urine culture. In these tests, a person's urine is examined for signs of disease. Most of the time in people with nocturnal enuresis, these test results come back completely normal.

How is it treated?

There are several things doctors can do to treat bedwetting, depending on what is causing it. If an illness is found to be the cause, which is not very common, it will be treated. If the history and physical examination do not suggest a specific medical problem, and the urine tests are negative, there are several behavioral approaches that can be used for treatment:

- Manage what you eat and drink before bed. People with nocturnal enuresis can take some basic steps to prevent an overfull bladder by decreasing the amount of fluids they drink before going to bed. Although you'll want to cut back on the amount of fluid you drink in the evening, no one should go to bed thirsty. You can reduce the chances that you'll wet the bed by going to the toilet just before bedtime.

> ✔ Quick Tip
> It may help to avoid eating certain foods in the evening: Foods that can irritate the bladder include coffee, tea, chocolate, and sodas or other carbonated beverages containing caffeine. And some people find that avoiding dairy foods at night may prevent the deep sleep that can contribute to enuresis.

- Imagine yourself dry. Using a technique called positive imagery, where you think about waking up dry before you go to sleep, can help some people stop bedwetting. Some people find that rewarding themselves for waking up dry also works.

- Use bedwetting alarms. Doctors and nurses sometimes prescribe bedwetting alarms to treat teens with enuresis. According to the National Kidney Foundation, 50% to 70% of cases of enuresis respond to treatment with these moisture alarms. With these alarms, a bell or buzzer goes off when a person begins to wet the bed. Then, you can quickly turn the alarm off, go to the toilet, and go back to sleep without wetting the bed too much. Don't get discouraged if the alarm doesn't help you stop wetting the bed immediately, though. It can take many weeks for the body to unlearn something it's been doing for years. Eventually, you can train yourself to get up before the alarm goes off or to hold your urine until morning.

People who sleep very deeply may need to rely on a parent or other family member to wake them up if they don't hear the alarm. The key to bedwetting alarms is waking up quickly—the sooner a person wakes up, the more effective the behavior modification for telling the brain to wake up or send the bladder signals to hold the urine until the morning.

Sometimes doctors treat enuresis with medication—although this is not usually the first course of action because no medication has been proven to cure bedwetting permanently, and the problem usually returns when the medication is stopped. In people whose bodies don't make enough ADH, doctors sometimes prescribe a man-made form of this hormone to decrease urine buildup during the night. Other medications relax the bladder, allowing it to hold more urine.

If you're worried about enuresis, the best thing to do is talk to your doctor for ideas on how to cope with it. Your mom or dad can also give you tips on how to cope, especially if he or she had the problem during adolescence. The good news is that scientists and doctors are learning more and more about bedwetting and are constantly developing new treatments for the problem.

Chapter 29

Bruxism

Do you ever wake up in the morning with a sore mouth or jaw? Have you ever slept over at a friend's house and been told, "You grind your teeth when you sleep"? If so, you might have bruxism.

What is bruxism?

Bruxism is the term for grinding or clenching your teeth. It comes from the Greek word "*brychein*," which means to grind or gnash the teeth. Bruxism can happen during the day, but it usually happens when you are asleep. Most of the time you don't even know you're doing it. It can happen to kids who still have all their baby teeth or kids whose permanent teeth are starting to grow in.

Dentists don't know for sure why some people grind their teeth, but they think it may have something to do with a person's bite—which means the way the top and bottom teeth fit together. Stress also may be behind bruxism. Have you ever worried about a test at school, something a bully said to you, or moving to a new town? Your body can react to these nervous feelings and fears in different ways, like grinding or clenching your teeth.

About This Chapter: This information, from "Taking the Bite Out of Bruxism," was provided by TeensHealth, one of the largest resources online for medically reviewed health information written for parents, kids, and teens. For more articles like this one, visit www.TeensHealth.org, or www.KidsHealth.org. © 2006 The Nemours Foundation.

Many kids grind their teeth at some time or another. Most of the time, it doesn't cause any pain or damage to your teeth. But if you share a room, you could drive your brother or sister nuts with the sound! In serious cases, nighttime grinding can wear down tooth enamel (the hard covering on your teeth) and cause jaw problems and pain. But these problems usually happen to grown-ups.

> ### ✎ What's It Mean?
>
> Bite: The way a person's top and bottom teeth fit together.
>
> Tooth Enamel: The hard covering on your teeth.

What will the dentist do?

You'll probably grow out of the teeth grinding. If it's making your jaw and face sore or giving you headaches, talk to your dentist. Your dentist will examine your teeth to see if the tooth enamel is worn down or chipped. The dentist also might ask questions about your teeth. For instance, the dentist might ask your parents if they hear you grinding your teeth when you're asleep.

Usually, kids don't need to do anything about bruxism. But if it's causing you pain or other problems, the dentist might give you something called a night guard. A night guard is a piece of plastic, kind of like a mouth guard that a football player wears. A night guard is worn at night and is fitted especially for your teeth and mouth to prevent you from grinding your teeth. Wearing one now can prevent problems later.

Goodbye To The Grinding

Because stress could be the cause of bruxism, you might try changing your bedtime routine so you're relaxed by the time you say good night. Take a warm bath or shower, listen to slow music, or read a good book. It just might help you say bye-bye to bruxism.

Chapter 30

Nocturnal Asthma

Asthma is a chronic condition in which the airways are hyperreactive (very sensitive) to certain irritants that cause them to constrict, thus making breathing difficult. This constriction (called bronchospasm) is accompanied by inflammation in the membranes lining the walls of the airways and excess production of mucus (phlegm).

The net effect has been described as a feeling that one is "breathing through a straw." Triggering irritants may include allergens, smoke, fumes, and dry, cold air. Exertion during exercise or even from laughing can also cause the airways to constrict. Asthmatics vary considerably in the severity of symptoms, response to treatment and the impact of illness on their lives.

Nighttime Worsening

Asthma symptoms can change a great deal during sleep. And although sleep-related asthma can occur at any time of the day, it is generally called "nocturnal asthma" since most people sleep at night. Nocturnal asthma is defined as any sleep-related worsening of reversible airway disease. Symptoms generally include shortness of breath or coughing and wheezing at night. Approximately 80 percent of severe asthmatic attacks occur between midnight and 8 A.M.

The Chronobiology Of Asthma

Many biological processes occur cycli-
cally. While some biological rhythms occur
monthly or annually, asthma changes fairly
predictably on a 24 hour or circadian cycle.

> ✎ **What's It Mean?**
> Chronobiology: The study
> of biological processes with
> time-related rhythms.

Lung function differs even in normal, non-asthmatics between day and
night. Optimal lung function occurs about 4 P.M. and poorest about 4 A.M. In
non-asthmatics, the difference is so insignificant that it goes unnoticed. But
in asthmatics, lung function can change as much as 50 percent over the course
of a day. Bronchial reactivity generally follows the same circadian cycle in
asthmatics—greatest reactivity corresponds with poorest lung function at 4
A.M. and lowest reactivity corresponds with optimal lung function at 4 P.M.

Changes in lung function at night are likely not due to the effects of lying
down. Studies show that lung function is related primarily to the time of day
or night a person sleeps. Thus, the rhythms are likely to be reversed in someone who works nights and sleeps days.

Causes Of Nocturnal Asthma

Nocturnal asthma is probably attributable to multiple, interactive factors
rather than to a single cause. Allergens are a major factor triggering asthma
attacks. Daytime exposure to allergens can be every bit as important as exposure to allergens in the bedroom during sleep. Allergens in the airways pre-
cipitate a series of physiological events as long as three to eight hours after
the initial exposure. This is called late-asthma response (LAR); it may correspond to the nighttime for some people and it can recur over several nights.
Allergen exposure in the evening increases a susceptible patient's risk of LAR
from 40 to 90 percent.

Asthma is an inflammatory disease. In certain people, this inflammation
worsens at night and tends to correspond with circadian changes in peak
expiratory flow rates (the ability to exhale rapidly). Airway secretions may be
a contributing factor to nocturnal asthma. About 70 percent of asthmatics
experience chronic sinusitis and/or postnasal drip. When the sinuses are
cleared, daytime and nighttime symptoms of asthma often improve.

Airway temperature also influences onset of symptoms. Even a brief exposure to cold, dry air can produce bronchospasm. The effect can be reversed by breathing warm, humidified air. Asthmatics may experience sleep apnea, characterized by brief, repetitive cessation of breathing during sleep. Resulting from an upper airway disturbance, sleep apnea triggers asthma of the lower airways.

Gastroesophageal reflux (GER) is a condition in which gastric acid "backs up" (refluxes) into the esophagus, resulting in "heartburn." GER is caused by a faulty valve that permits the reflux of stomach contents. A variation of this condition may trigger nocturnal asthma. When a person with a faulty valve lies flat, gravity may allow for a small amount of acid to reflux far enough to be inhaled into the airway, triggering bronchospasm.

Certain hormones and other body chemicals are involved in the relaxation of smooth muscle and the cellular response leading to asthma. Circadian changes in these chemicals correlate with noted changes in lung function, but the significance of these changes is currently unclear.

Diagnosis Of Nocturnal Asthma

It is important to inform your clinician if asthma symptoms worsen at night. You may be asked to monitor your lung function using a peak flow meter. This is a portable device that measures the lung volume and how quickly air can be expelled from the lungs. Decreasing values measured by the peak flow meter indicate a tightening of the airways, and can serve as an early warning of impending respiratory symptoms, such as shortness of breath and wheezing. Nocturnal asthma can be documented by recording peak flow rates at bedtime, during any awakening at night and in the morning. The readings provide an objective basis for treatment; swings in peak flow rates help indicate persons at-risk of respiratory arrest, which occurs mostly at night.

Treatment

An understanding of the circadian rhythms of asthma and the effects of various medications enables your clinician to apply the concepts of chronopharmacology—the science of precisely timed drug administration. The primary principle is to apply the most intense therapy when the disease worsens.

An inhalant drug called Serevent, (salmeterol) provides sustained effectiveness against bronchoconstriction and is therefore the treatment of choice for prevention of nocturnal asthma attacks. Anti-inflammatory inhalants may also be useful.

Corticosteroid medications are potent anti-inflammatories that are occasionally used in cases of severe asthma. Inhaled steroids are preferable to oral steroids because they present fewer side effects. However, severe nocturnal asthma may indicate the use of oral steroid medication in the evening.

Treatments that improve sinusitis, if present, can also improve nocturnal asthma. Nasal irrigation, oral decongestants, and nasal steroids can reduce or eliminate upper airway inflammation and the consequent bronchoconstriction.

If sleep apnea is present, the clinician may suggest a variety of interventions, including a change in sleeping position, medications or a mechanical device that keeps the back of the throat open to prevent apnea. This device is called a nasal Continuous Positive Airway Pressure (CPAP). Asthmatics who experience gastroesophageal reflux (GER) are advised to raise their upper body so they sleep at a 45 degree angle. This prevents gravity from permitting acid reflux. Your clinician may also prescribe certain medications for GER.

☞ Remember!!

If you experience signs of nocturnal asthma, be sure to inform your clinician. Remember that asthma is a reversible disease that can be managed well with proper medical supervision.

Part Four

The Consequences Of Sleep Deprivation

Chapter 31

Sleep Deprivation May Be Undermining Teen Health

On any given school day, teen-agers across the nation stumble out of bed and prepare for the day. For most, the alarm clock buzzes by 6:30 A.M., a scant seven hours after they went to bed. Many students board the school bus before 7 A.M. and are in class by 7:30.

In adults, such meager sleep allowances are known to affect day-to-day functioning in myriad ways. In adolescents, who are biologically driven to sleep longer and later than adults do, the effects of insufficient sleep are likely to be even more dramatic—so much so that some sleep experts contend that the nation's early high-school start times, increasingly common, are tantamount to abuse.

"Almost all teen-agers, as they reach puberty, become walking zombies because they are getting far too little sleep," comments Cornell University psychologist James B. Maas, PhD, one of the nation's leading sleep experts.

There can be little question that sleep deprivation has negative effects on adolescents. According to the National Highway Traffic Safety Administration,

✤ It's A Fact!!

Lack of sufficient sleep—a rampant problem among teens—appears to put adolescents at risk for cognitive and emotional difficulties, poor school performance, accidents and psychopathology, research suggests.

Source: Carpenter, S. (2001). Sleep Deprivation May Be Undermining Teen Health. *Monitor on Psychology*, 32, 9.

for example, drowsiness and fatigue cause more than 100,000 traffic accidents each year—and young drivers are at the wheel in more than half of these crashes.

Insufficient sleep has also been shown to cause difficulties in school, including disciplinary problems, sleepiness in class and poor concentration.

"What good does it do to try to educate teen-agers so early in the morning?" asks Maas. "You can be giving the most stimulating, interesting lectures to sleep-deprived kids early in the morning or right after lunch, when they're at their sleepiest, and the overwhelming drive to sleep replaces any chance of alertness, cognition, memory, or understanding."

Recent research has also revealed an association between sleep deprivation and poorer grades. In a 1998 survey of more than 3,000 high-school students, for example, psychologists Amy R. Wolfson, PhD, of the College of the Holy Cross, and Mary A. Carskadon, PhD, of Brown University Medical School, found that students who reported that they were getting Cs, Ds and Fs in school obtained about 25 minutes less sleep and went to bed about 40 minutes later than students who reported they were getting As and Bs.

In August [2001], researchers at the University of Minnesota reported the results of a study of more than 7,000 high-school students whose school district had switched in 1997 from a 7:15 A.M. start time to an 8:40 A.M. start time. Compared with students whose schools maintained earlier start times, students with later starts reported getting more sleep on school nights, being less sleepy during the day, getting slightly higher grades, and experiencing fewer depressive feelings and behaviors.

Also troubling are findings that adolescent sleep difficulties are often associated with psychopathologies such as depression and attention deficit hyperactivity disorder (ADHD).

This research, combined with studies showing widespread sleep deprivation among teens, has propelled efforts to educate children and adults about the importance of a good night's sleep and to persuade schools to push back high-school starting times.

"There is substantial evidence that the lack of sleep can cause accidents, imperil students' grades, and lead to or exacerbate emotional problems," says U.S. Rep. Zoe Lofgren (D-Calif.), who has introduced a bill that would provide federal grants to help school districts defray the cost of pushing back school starting times. Adjusting school schedules, Lofgren says, "could do more to improve education and reduce teen accidents and crime than many more expensive initiatives."

♣ **It's A Fact!!**

What are the consequences of sleep deprivation?

• Motor vehicle accidents and work accidents

• Decreased productivity

• If this becomes a chronic problem, sleep deprivation can cause difficulties with social relationships because of irritability; as well as some significant medical problems.

Source: Excerpted from "Sleep Deprivation: Causes and Consequences," Nebraska Rural Health and Safety Coalition, © 2002 University of Nebraska Medical Center; reprinted with permission.

The research has also spurred further investigations into why teens need extra sleep, the effects of sleep deprivation on cognition, emotion regulation and psychopathology, and the long-term consequences of chronic sleep deprivation.

Dogma Reversed

For decades, experts believed that people require less sleep as they move from infancy through adulthood.

It's easy to see why this belief persisted: Adolescents sleep less than they did as children, declining from an average of 10 hours a night during middle childhood to fewer than 7.5 hours by age 16. According to Wolfson and Carskadon's 1998 study,

26 percent of high school students routinely sleep less than 6.5 hours on school nights, and only 15 percent sleep 8.5 hours or more. The same study indicated that to make up for lost sleep, most teens snooze an extra couple of hours on weekend mornings—a habit that can lead to poorer-quality sleep.

But to researchers' surprise, in the past two decades studies have shown that teen-agers require considerably more sleep to perform optimally than do younger children or adults. Starting around the beginning of puberty and continuing into their early 20s, Carskadon and colleagues have shown, adolescents need about 9.2 hours of sleep each night, compared with the 7.5 to 8 hours that adults need.

♣ **It's A Fact!!**
When are accidents related to sleep deprivation most likely to happen?

• In the early to mid afternoon and in the very early morning hours. These are the times when everyone is least alert.

Source: Excerpted from "Sleep Deprivation: Causes and Consequences," Nebraska Rural Health and Safety Coalition, © 2002 University of Nebraska Medical Center; reprinted with permission.

In addition to needing more sleep, adolescents experience a "phase shift" during puberty, falling asleep later at night than do younger children. Researchers long assumed that this shift was driven by psychosocial factors such as social activities, academic pressures, evening jobs, and television and internet use. In the past several years, however, sleep experts have learned that biology also plays a starring role in adolescents' changing sleep patterns, says Carskadon.

Indeed, Carskadon's research is greatly responsible for that new understanding. In a pair of groundbreaking studies published in 1993 and 1997, she and colleagues found that more physically mature girls preferred activities later in the day than did less mature girls, and that in more physically mature teens, melatonin production tapered off later than it did in less mature teens. Those findings, Carskadon says, suggest that the brain's circadian timing system—controlled mainly by melatonin—switches on later at night as pubertal development progresses.

Changes in adolescents' circadian timing system, combined with external pressures such as the need to awaken early in the morning for school, produce a potentially destructive pattern of early-morning sleepiness in teenagers, Carskadon argues. In a laboratory study of 40 high-school students published in the journal *Sleep* (Vol. 21, No. 8) in 1998, she, Wolfson, and colleagues examined the effect of changing school starting times from 8:25 A.M. to 7:20 A.M.

Their results were disturbing: Almost half of the students who began school at 7:20 were "pathologically sleepy" at 8:30, falling directly into REM sleep in an average of only 3.4 minutes—a pattern similar to what is seen in patients with narcolepsy.

Those findings, says Carskadon, persuaded her that "these early school start times are just abusive. These kids may be up and at school at 8:30, but I'm convinced their brains are back on the pillow at home."

Elusive Questions

The evidence of adolescents' increased need for sleep and that many— if not most—teen-agers are chronically sleep deprived has raised further questions. Particularly elusive, says Carskadon, has been the question of why adolescents' circadian clocks shift to a later phase around the beginning of puberty.

One possibility, she believes, is that the brain's sensitivity to light changes during adolescence. At the annual meeting of the Associated Professional Sleep Societies in June [2001], she and colleagues presented research showing that in the evening, exposure to even very dim lighting delayed melatonin secretion for participants who were in middle or late puberty, but not for prepubertal participants.

Carskadon is also interested in how teen-age alcohol use might affect the brain's sleep system. Following up on studies in adults that have established a link between drinking problems and changes in sleep patterns, for example, she and her colleagues plan to examine whether during early development, young people with a family history of problem drinking might have abnormalities in the brain mechanisms that govern sleep.

♣ It's A Fact!!
Epworth Sleepiness Scale

Name:

Today's date:

Your age (Yrs):

Your sex (Male = M, Female = F):

How likely are you to doze off or fall asleep in the following situations, in contrast to feeling just tired? This refers to your usual way of life in recent times. Even if you haven't done some of these things recently try to work out how they would have affected you.

Use the following scale to choose the most appropriate number for each situation:

0 = would **never** doze

1 = **slight chance** of dozing

2 = **moderate chance** of dozing

3 = **high chance** of dozing

It is important that you answer each question as best you can.

Situation	**Chance of Dozing (0-3)**
Sitting and reading	_____
Watching TV	_____
Sitting, inactive in a public place (e.g. a theatre or a meeting)	_____
As a passenger in a car for an hour without a break	_____
Lying down to rest in the afternoon when circumstances permit	_____
Sitting and talking to someone	_____
Sitting quietly after a lunch without alcohol	_____
In a car, while stopped for a few minutes in the traffic	_____

Source: "Epworth Sleepiness Scale," © MW Johns 1990-97, reproduced with permission.

Just as important as the question of why sleep patterns change during adolescence is the issue of how sleep deprivation influences adolescents' emotion regulation and behavior. Many researchers have noted that sleep-deprived teen-agers appear to be especially vulnerable to psychopathologies such as depression and ADHD, and to have difficulty controlling their emotions and impulses.

Although it's difficult to untangle cause and effect, it's likely that sleep deprivation and problems controlling impulses and emotions exacerbate one another, leading to a "negative spiral" of fatigue and sleepiness, labile emotions, poor decision-making, and risky behavior, says Ronald E. Dahl, MD, a professor of psychiatry and pediatrics at the University of Pittsburgh.

Despite the evidence that insufficient sleep affects young people's thinking, emotional balance, and behavior, the long-term effects of chronic sleep deprivation on learning, emotion, social relationships, and health remain uncertain.

"There's a real need for longitudinal studies to follow through later childhood and adulthood," says psychologist Avi Sadeh, PhD, a sleep researcher at Tel Aviv University. Although research has amply demonstrated that sleep problems affect young people's cognitive skills, behavior and temperament in the short term, he says, "It's not at all clear to what extent these effects are long-lasting."

✔ Quick Tip
Scoring the Epworth Sleepiness Scale

The Epworth Sleepiness Scale (ESS) score is the sum of the eight numbers given as answers to the questions. This score can vary between 0 and 24. A score greater than 10 indicates significant excessive daytime sleepiness.

Source: "Epworth Sleepiness Scale," © MW Johns 1990-97, reproduced with permission.

Researchers Push For School Changes, Public Outreach

With such a wealth of evidence about the prevalence of adolescent sleep deprivation and the risks it poses, many sleep researchers have become involved in efforts to persuade school districts to push back high-school starting times so that teens can get their needed rest.

Some schools argue that adjusting school schedules is too expensive and complicated. But others have responded positively to sleep experts' pleas. The Connecticut legislature is considering a bill that would prohibit public schools from starting before 8:30 A.M., and Massachusetts lawmakers are also weighing the issue. And Lofgren's "Zzzzz's to A's" bill, first introduced in the U.S. House of Representatives in 1998, would provide federal grants of up to $25,000 to school districts to help cover the administrative costs of adjusting school start times.

These efforts are a move in the right direction, says Wolfson. But, she says, changing school start times isn't the entire answer. "I think we have to be educating children, parents, and teachers about the importance of sleep, just as we educate them about exercise, nutrition, and drug and alcohol use."

Toward that end, several public-education efforts are now under way:

• With a grant from the Simmons mattress company, Cornell's Maas recently produced a film on teen-age sleep deprivation, its consequences and the "golden rules" for healthy sleep. The film is scheduled for distribution through parent-teacher associations and school principals this fall [2001]. In August [2001], Maas also published a children's book, "Remmy and the Brain Train," which discusses why the brain requires a good night's sleep.

• Next year [2002], the National Center for Sleep Disorders Research at the National Institutes of Health plans to release a supplemental sleep curriculum for 10th-grade biology classes, addressing the biology of sleep, the consequences of insufficient sleep and the major sleep disorders. In a related effort, the center is coordinating a sleep-education campaign aimed at 7- to 11-year-olds.

- Wolfson and colleague Christine A. Marco, PhD, a psychologist at Worcester State College, are pilot-testing an eight-week sleep curriculum for middle-school students. As part of the curriculum, students keep sleep diaries, play creative games, and participate in role-playing about sleep, and set goals—for example, for the amount of sleep they want to get or for regulating their caffeine intake. Preliminary results indicate that the curriculum helps students improve their sleep habits.

"Changing school start times is one critical measure we can take to protect young people's sleep," says Wolfson. "And then, if we can only understand what's going on with sleep in these sixth-, seventh- and eighth-graders, we can intervene to change their sleep behavior before it gets out of hand."

Chapter 32

Is It Attention Deficit Hyperactivity Disorder Or Sleep Deprivation?

Feeling moody, restless or unable to concentrate is no way to go through life, so most teens who feel this way want to know what they can do about it! Sleep deprivation makes it difficult to learn and can lead to inattention or difficulty controlling impulsive, emotional reactions to situations. These are some of the same symptoms, however, that can lead to a diagnosis of attention deficit hyperactivity disorder (ADHD), so it is important to include sleep in the overall picture when evaluating any difficulties you may be having.

ADHD is a distinct disorder; however, research has shown that some people may be misdiagnosed with ADHD when the real problem is chronic sleep deprivation, due to a sleep disorder or poor sleeping habits. In addition, studies show that many people with ADHD also suffer from sleep disorders such as sleep apnea, insomnia, or restless legs syndrome. In many cases, people who have both ADHD and a sleep disorder have shown marked improvement in their symptoms after the sleep problem is treated.

When teens either show symptoms of ADHD or are diagnosed with it, a sleep assessment should be included as part of the overall picture. Before meeting with your doctor, it may help to keep a sleep diary for two weeks and bring it with you to your appointment. Be prepared to discuss:

Sleep Habits And/Or Problems

- Difficulty falling asleep or staying asleep

- Difficulty waking in the morning

- Snoring, gasping for breath, or pauses in breathing during sleep

- Restless sleep

- Any known sleep disorders, such as insomnia, sleep apnea, restless legs syndrome, or a circadian rhythm disorder

- Medical conditions that may interfere with your sleep, including obesity, upper airway obstruction, pain, neurological, or psychiatric conditions

- Medications you are taking that may be disrupting your sleep

- Sleep environment and possible disruptive factors

- Lifestyle factors that may contribute to sleep deprivation, such as overextending yourself with schoolwork, sports, clubs, social activities, part-time jobs, and family obligations

> ### ✔ Quick Tip
>
> It is important that you tell your doctor about the duration and severity of your symptoms, as well as other strategies you have used to cope with them. Ensuring that you are getting enough sleep is crucial, and a sleep study can help if a sleep disorder is suspected. Since people with ADHD often have unstable sleep-wake patterns—sleeping well some nights and poorly others—the sleep study may be more effective if it evaluates sleep over several consecutive nights to reveal the overall sleep pattern. Whether a sleep disturbance is the root cause of the problem or not, it is important to talk to your doctor about sleep, since any treatment should go hand in hand with good sleeping habits.

Daytime Symptoms

- Sleepiness

- Declining performance in school and other activities

- Difficulty paying attention

- Mood or personality changes

- Memory problems

- Physical complaints (for example, headaches)

What Are The Symptoms Of ADHD?

The *Diagnostic and Statistical Manual* (*DSM-IV*) divides ADHD into three types: inattentiveness, hyperactivity/impulsivity, and combined. To be diagnosed with ADHD, a person should meet A–E of the following criteria:

A: Either 1 or 2:

1. Six or more of the following symptoms of inattention have persisted for at least six months to a degree that is maladaptive and inconsistent with developmental level:

   • Often fails to give close attention to details or makes careless mistakes in schoolwork, work, or other activities

   • Often has difficulty sustaining attention in tasks or play activities

   • Often does not seem to listen when spoken to directly

   • Often does not follow through on instructions and fails to finish school-work, chores, or duties in the workplace (not due to oppositional behavior or failure to understand instructions)

   • Often has difficulty organizing tasks and activities

   • Often avoids, dislikes, or is reluctant to engage in tasks that require sustained mental effort (such as homework)

   • Often loses things necessary for tasks or activities (toys, school assignments, pencils, books, or tools)

   • Is often easily distracted by extraneous stimuli

   • Is often forgetful in daily activities

2. Six or more of the following symptoms of hyperactivity-impulsivity have persisted for at least six months to a degree that is maladaptive and inconsistent with developmental level:

   • Often fidgets with hands or feet or squirms in seat

   • Often leaves seat in classroom or in other situations in which remaining seated is expected

- Often runs about or climbs excessively in situations in which it is inappropriate (in adolescents or adults, may be limited to subjective feelings of restlessness)

- Often has difficulty playing or engaging in leisure activities quietly

- Is often "on the go" or often acts as if "driven by a motor"

- Often talks excessively

- Often blurts out answers before questions have been completed

- Often has difficulty awaiting turn

- Often interrupts or intrudes on others (such as butting into conversations or games)

B: Some hyperactive, impulsive, or inattentive symptoms that caused impairment were present before age 7 years.

C: Some impairment from the symptoms is present in two or more settings (such as in school or work and at home).

D: There must be clear evidence of clinically significant impairment in social, academic, or occupational functioning.

E: The symptoms do not occur exclusively during the course of a pervasive developmental disorder, schizophrenia, or another psychotic disorder and are not better accounted for by another mental disorder.

Chapter 33

Teens, Sleep Deprivation, And Depression

What You Should Know About Teens, Sleep, And Depression

- Over the past two weeks, have you felt down, depressed, or hopeless?

- Over the past two weeks, have you felt little interest or pleasure in doing things?

Scientists on the U.S. Preventive Services Task Force recommended in 2002 that doctors ask these two questions to screen their patients for depression. Since depression may go unrecognized or be misdiagnosed, it can help to know common signs of both depression and other problems that may cause similar symptoms.

Both depression and sleep deprivation can interfere with our ability to think, work, socialize, and enjoy life. Both have a number of symptoms in common. These include lack of energy, difficulty concentrating and making decisions, moody behavior, unusual sleep patterns, loss of interest in activities, as well as weight and appetite changes. In addition, interrupted sleep is very common among people who are depressed. Over 90% of those with depression complain about difficulty falling asleep, frequent nighttime awakenings and early morning awakenings. Others may sleep much more than usual and still feel tired.

Teens need at least 8½ hours—and on average 9¼ hours—of sleep each night to function at their best. In addition, biological sleep patterns shift toward later times for both sleeping and waking during adolescence, so it is natural to not be able to fall asleep before 11:00 P.M. or later. Teens also tend to have irregular sleep patterns across the week—they typically stay up late and sleep in late on the weekends, which can affect their biological clocks and hurt the quality of their sleep. Some teens experience sleep problems such as sleep apnea and insomnia, which keep them from getting the sleep they need. These factors during adolescence can contribute to sleep deprivation in teens, which can greatly impact performance in school and other areas, as well as overall quality of life.

It is normal for teens to have times when they feel tired, sad, moody, or have difficulty focusing on school and other important things in their lives. If these feelings linger, intensify, and begin to interfere with life at school and at home, however, it may be time to talk with your doctor to find an appropriate treatment.

Symptoms that may indicate depression include:

- feeling persistently sad, anxious, hopeless or empty for several weeks, months or longer;

- sleeping more or less than usual;

- loss of interest in things you used to like and enjoy;

- lack of energy;

- weight changes and appetite disturbances;

- moodiness;

- feeling guilty, helpless, or worthless;

- difficulty concentrating, remembering things, and making decisions;

♣ **It's A Fact!!**

Most people who are depressed do not commit suicide. But depression increases the risk for suicide or suicide attempts. It is not true that people who talk about suicide do not attempt it. Suicidal thoughts, remarks, or attempts are always serious. If any of these happen to you or a friend, you must tell a responsible adult immediately. It's better to be safe than sorry.

Source: Excerpted from "Let's Talk About Depression," National Institute of Mental Health, updated February 2006.

- withdrawal from friends or family;

- loss of self-confidence and self-esteem;

- irritability and restlessness;

- frequent complaints of headaches, stomach aches, or other pains;

- doing poorly in school;

- thoughts of death and suicide.

Depression is an illness that involves the body, mood, and thoughts. About one out of 12 teenagers suffers from depression before the age of eighteen. Half of the teenagers who go untreated for depression may attempt suicide, which is the third leading cause of death among teens. While it can disrupt life by affecting a person's ability to function, relate well to others, and experience pleasure, it is a treatable illness.

Insomnia And Depression: Are They Related?

The most common sleep disorder related to depression is insomnia. In a Johns Hopkins University study of 1,000 young male medical students, researchers found that insomnia might be a predictive factor for later episodes of severe depression and other types of serious mental disorders. Insomnia is a risk factor for the onset of depression and can significantly affect quality of life. While some studies indicate insomnia as a trigger for depression, insomnia can also show up as symptom once depression occurs. In fact, depression is considered one of the most prevalent causes of insomnia.

Insomnia symptoms include:

- difficulty falling asleep;

- difficulty staying asleep;

- waking too early in the morning;

- experiencing non-restorative sleep.

If teens feel they are experiencing symptoms of depression or a sleep disorder, they should talk to a doctor, and may find it useful to keep a journal of symptoms and sleep patterns to discuss at the appointment.

✔ Quick Tip

Here's how to tell if you or a friend might be depressed.

First, there are two kinds of depressive illness: the sad kind, called major depression, and manic-depression or bipolar disorder, when feeling down and depressed alternates with being speeded-up and sometimes reckless.

You should get evaluated by a professional if you've had five or more of the following symptoms for more than two weeks or if any of these symptoms cause such a big change that you can't keep up your usual routine:

When You're Depressed

- You feel sad or cry a lot and it doesn't go away.

- You feel guilty for no reason; you feel like you're no good; you've lost your confidence.

- Life seems meaningless or like nothing good is ever going to happen again. You have a negative attitude a lot of the time, or it seems like you have no feelings.

- You don't feel like doing a lot of the things you used to like—like music, sports, being with friends, going out—and you want to be left alone most of the time.

- It's hard to make up your mind. You forget lots of things, and it's hard to concentrate.

- You get irritated often. Little things make you lose your temper; you over-react.

- Your sleep pattern changes; you start sleeping a lot more or you have trouble falling asleep at night. Or you wake up really early most mornings and can't get back to sleep.

- Your eating pattern changes; you've lost your appetite or you eat a lot more.

- You feel restless and tired most of the time.

- You think about death, or feel like you're dying, or have thoughts about committing suicide.

When You're Manic

- You feel high as a kite...like you're "on top of the world."

- You get unreal ideas about the great things you can do...things that you really can't do.

- Thoughts go racing through your head, you jump from one subject to another, and you talk a lot.

- You're a non-stop party, constantly running around.

- You do too many wild or risky things: with driving, with spending money, with sex, etc.

- You're so "up" that you don't need much sleep.

- You're rebellious or irritable and can't get along at home or school, or with your friends.

Talk To Someone

If you are concerned about depression in yourself or a friend, talk to someone about it. There are people who can help you get treatment:

- a professional at a mental health center or Mental Health Association

- a trusted family member

- your family doctor

- your clergy

- a school counselor or nurse

- a social worker

- a responsible adult

Or, if you don't know where to turn, the telephone directory or information operator should have phone numbers for a local hotline or mental health services or referrals.

Source: Excerpted from "Let's Talk About Depression," National Institute of Mental Health, updated February 2006.

Adolescent Moods And Sleep

When It's More Than Just Waking Up On The Wrong Side Of The Bed

While everyone is accustomed to having a bad morning here and there—feeling irritable, unhappy, or even sad, the National Sleep Foundation (NSF)'s 2006 Sleep in America poll found that many adolescents exhibit symptoms of a depressive mood on a frequent if not daily basis, and these teens are more likely to have sleep problems.

The NSF poll calculated depressive mood scores for each of the 1,602 poll respondents by measuring adolescents' responses to four mood states (using a scale of "1" to "3" where 1 equals "not at all" and 3 equals "much"):

• Felt unhappy, sad or depressed;

• Felt hopeless about the future;

• Felt nervous or tense; and

• Worried too much about things.

The results showed that about half (46%) of the adolescents surveyed had a depressive mood score of 10 to 14, 37% had a score of 15 to 19, and 17% had a score of 20 to 30; these scores are considered low, moderate, and high respectively.

Most notably, those adolescents with high scores ranging from 20 to 30 were more likely than those with lower scores to take longer to fall asleep on school nights, get an insufficient amount of sleep, and have sleep problems related to sleepiness. In fact, 73% of those adolescents who report feeling unhappy, sad, or depressed also report not getting enough sleep at night and being excessively sleepy during the day.

While many adults may think that adolescents have things easy or don't have much to worry about—the opposite seems true according to the NSF poll. Most adolescents were likely to say they worried about things too much (58%) and/or felt stressed out/anxious (56%). Many of the adolescents surveyed also reported feeling hopeless about the future, or feeling unhappy, sad, or depressed much or somewhat within the past two weeks of surveying.

Research shows that lack of sleep affects mood, and a depressed mood can lead to lack of sleep. To combat this vicious cycle, sleep experts recommend that teens prioritize sleep and focus on healthy sleep habits. Teens can start by getting the 8½ to 9¼ hours of sleep they need each night, keeping consistent sleep and wake schedules on school nights and weekends, and opting for relaxing activities such as reading or taking a warm shower or bath before bed instead of turning on the TV or computer.

"If parents and teens know what good sleep entails and the benefits of making and sticking to a plan that supports good sleep, then they might re-examine their choices about what truly are their 'essential' activities," says Mary Carskadon, Ph.D., Director of Chronobiology/Sleep Research at the E.P. Bradley Hospital and Professor of Psychiatry and Human Behavior at Brown Medical School in Providence, R.I. "The earlier parents can start helping their children with good sleep habits, the easier it will be to sustain them through the teen years."

☞ Remember!!

- Depression is a real medical illness and it's treatable.

- Depression is more than just being moody, and it can affect people at any age, including teenagers.

- Depression, which saps energy and self-esteem, interferes with a person's ability or wish to get help. It is an act of true friendship to share your concerns with an adult who can help.

- Talking through feelings with a good friend is often a helpful first step. Friendship, concern, and support can provide the encouragement to talk to a parent or other trusted adult about getting evaluated for depression.

Source: Excerpted from "Let's Talk About Depression," National Institute of Mental Health, updated February 2006.

Chapter 34

Sleep Deprivation Affects Sports Performance

Sleep And Sports: Get The Winning Edge!

"Ready, hike!" He sprints towards the end zone, glancing over his shoulder as he waits for the ball to come sailing through the air towards him. The further he goes, the more tired he feels. He sees the ball launched into the air heading his way. He steps over the line into the end zone. The ball has almost reached him. Here it comes. Splat! The ball fell right through his hands. This could happen to you.

If you are experiencing sleep deprivation, your athletic performance may suffer. Sleep deprivation does not mean you pulled an all-nighter. Building a cumulative sleep debt, getting less than the 9¼ hours of sleep you need per night, can produce the same results in as little as two weeks. Given that 85% of teens get less than 8½ hours of sleep per night, our star quarterback is probably suffering from sleep deprivation and stifling his true athletic potential.

Some effects of sleep deprivation on sports performance are physiological, which means they happen in the body. These can include:

- Impaired motor function, which can include tremors, incoordination, blurred vision, and/or prolonged reaction time. In fact, reaction time has been shown to be equally slowed in sleep-deprived individuals as those who are legally drunk.

♣ It's A Fact!!
Sleep Reorganizes Brain Connections
To Improve Performance

Sleep helps strengthen memories and improves physical performance by producing large-scale changes in brain activity that makes a skill less dependent on conscious thought, Dr. Matthew P. Walker and colleagues at Harvard Medical School has found. Twelve healthy, college-aged participants were taught a simple finger-tapping task and then retested 12 hours later, either after a night of sleep or after 12 daytime hours without sleep. The researchers monitored the participants' brain activity using functional magnetic resonance imaging (fMRI). Those who slept performed the task with fewer errors than those in the daytime test group, and showed greater brain activation in the motor cortex and cerebellum (which control speed and accuracy) as well as in the right frontal lobe and right temporal lobe (which help create memory sequences). This increased activation suggests that sleep reinforced the memory of the task in motor control areas of the brain, allowing participants to perform the task more quickly and accurately. In addition, those who slept showed decreased brain activity in the parietal lobes (involved in conscious monitoring of physical movement) and several emotion-regulating regions, suggesting that as memory of the task was reinforced it became easier to perform without thinking about it too much. This, in turn, may have reduced the emotional burden involved in performing the task. The researchers propose that further studies are needed to find out whether a full night of sleep prompts these changes in the brain, or whether they are triggered by a specific stage of sleep. Such findings have important implications not only for learning real-life skills (such as learning a musical instrument or playing a sport), but also for physical rehabilitation (such as after a stroke), and for studying the relationship between sleep disturbances and learning problems.

Reference: Walker MP, Stickgold R, Alsop D, Gaab N, Schlaug G. Sleep-dependent motor memory plasticity in the human brain. *Neuroscience*. 2005. 133(4):911-917.

Source: From "Science Updates, 2005," National Institute of Mental Health (www.nimh.nih.gov), 2005.

- Delayed visual reaction time so that by the time you see the ball heading toward you, it could hit you in the head.

- Delayed auditory reaction time means that you may not hear your teammate calling to you until it is too late.

- Reduced cardiovascular performance can mean that your fitness may be down by as much as 11%.

- Diminished mental functioning can occur so that you will not be able to remember the plays you learned at practice yesterday.

- Reduced endurance which means that you may get tired sooner because glucose storage is slowed with sleep deprivation.

Some of the effects are emotional or psychological. These can be equally harmful to your performance at a big game. They include:

- **Increased Perceived Exertion:** Even if you can physically perform at similar levels, you will feel tired more quickly and give up.

- **Impaired Moods:** Sleep deprivation can leave you in a bad mood; you'll certainly not be at the top mental state you need for a championship match.

On the positive side, getting enough sleep will actually help you to learn new physical skills. Studies have shown that sleep builds procedural memory, so you'll remember the plays you trained for over and over at practice. Motor skills continue to be learned as you sleep. You will notice an improvement the next day, even if you have not practiced since.

Your body works very hard every day to keep up with all of the things that you do. You put it through a grueling day at school, a few hours of homework, and if you add athletics on top of that, you are really pushing the limits of your body. Sleep is absolutely essential to maintaining a level of success in all of these activities, as well as in your relationships, health and appearance.

So, get your sleep and score big.

Sleep May Be Athletes' Best Performance Booster

Text under this heading is from "Sleep May Be Athletes' Best Performance Booster," by Lynne Lamberg, *Psychiatric News*, August 19, 2005. Reprinted with permission from *Psychiatric News*, Copyright © 2005 American Psychiatric Association.

Athlete A or team X, the top performers in their sport, sometimes lose to less-adept competitors. Lower-ranked athletes or teams, at their peak, may perform better than top-ranked ones at their worst. Even elite athletes aren't always at the top of their game.

Variations in sports performance may reflect normal ebb and flow of biological rhythms. Marked differences between time of training and time of competition—as commonly occur in figure skating and football—also may dent an athlete's performance, noted Teodor Postolache, M.D., an associate professor of psychiatry at the University of Maryland School of Medicine.

> ✤ **It's A Fact!!**
> Chronobiology studies are giving athletes and coaches valuable information on sleep strategies that could help ensure that an athlete's performance doesn't become a victim of too little sleep.
>
> Source: Copyright © 2005 American Psychiatric Association.

Postolache served as guest editor of the June [2005] *Clinics in Sports Medicine*, which explores applications of body-time research to sports performance. (This issue was published as a book, *Sports Chronobiology*, by Saunders.)

Normal mid-afternoon drowsiness, jet travel, seasonal and menstrual-cycle variations in body rhythms, and lack of sleep can take the edge off athletic skills, Postolache said. Chronobiology lab findings can help athletes perform at their peak and reduce their risk of injury.

Psychiatrists and psychologists working in medical school psychiatry departments report their research in some of the book's 18 articles.

Psychomotor Vigilance Declines

Hans Van Dongen, Ph.D., and David Dinges, Ph.D., of the University of Pennsylvania, described studies assessing psychomotor vigilance performance after sleep deprivation. This skill involves reaction time and sustained attention. It is needed for not only sports performance but also everyday activities such as driving. It is highly sensitive to sleep loss, often experienced by athletes on road trips, particularly after they cross multiple time zones.

Such performance deteriorates markedly after 88 hours of continuous wakefulness, a duration comparable to staying up for three nights and long enough to show circadian patterns of alertness and sleepiness. Performance is consistently better in the day than at night, a reflection of humans' innate programming to stay alert in the day and sleep at night. Two-hour nap opportunities every 12 hours can blunt deficits in psychomotor vigilance.

Naps have a downside, though. Right after awakening, people often manifest performance deficits termed "sleep inertia." They're foggy and clumsy. This effect intensifies with progressive sleep loss, especially at night, Van Dongen and Dinges found. Very short naps—roughly 10 minutes—may offer some recuperative benefit when people are sleep deprived, they said, without producing noticeable levels of sleep inertia.

'Sleep Debt' Snowballs

Chronic sleep restriction, widespread among American adults, has serious adverse consequences for physical and mental performance, asserted sleep researcher William Dement, M.D., Ph.D., a professor of psychiatry at Stanford University. The most important aspect of the body's homeostatic regulation of sleep, he said, is that sleep loss is cumulative. "When total nightly sleep is reduced by exactly the same amount each night for several consecutive nights," he reported, "the tendency to fall asleep in the daytime becomes progressively stronger each day."

Dement calls this phenomenon "sleep debt." As he explains, the brain records as a debt every hour of sleep that is less than a person's nightly requirement. This snowballing debt may include an hour of sleep lost a week or month ago, as well as the hour lost last night, he speculated. A large sleep debt can be reduced only by extra sleep.

In a landmark 1994 National Institute of Mental Health study, subjects stayed in bed in the dark 14 hours every night for 28 consecutive nights. At first, they slept as long as 12 hours a night, suggesting they entered the study with sizable sleep debts, Dement said. By the fourth week, their sleep stabilized at a nightly average of eight hours and 15 minutes—a figure interpreted to mean that most adults need this amount of sleep each night.

Does 'Secret' Advantage Accrue?

When subjects slept until "slept out," their mood, energy level, and sense of well-being as indicated on daily questionnaires all improved. Athletes who obtain all the sleep they need, Dement suggested, might have a "secret" advantage over their competition.

> **☞ Remember!!**
>
> Athletes who obtain all the sleep they need might have a "secret' advantage over their competition.
>
> Source: Copyright © 2005 American Psychiatric Association.

The adage "practice makes perfect," long a truism of athletic training, has been modified by sleep and chronobiology studies in the past decade, according to Matthew Walker, Ph.D., and Robert Stickgold, Ph.D., of Harvard Medical School. After initial training, the human brain continues to learn in the absence of further practice, they said. The improvement develops in sleep.

These findings have a direct application to athletes' training schedules, they asserted. Athletes who train consistently across the day and then cut short their sleep to get up early the next morning for practice might shortchange their brains of sleep-dependent consolidation and plasticity.

Studies of bright light's beneficial impact on mood hold relevance for the depressed athlete who experiences adverse effects from antidepressant medications or needs to avoid psychoactive substances entirely, said Postolache and Dan Oren, M.D., of Yale University School of Medicine. Bright light's antidepressant effects start sooner than those of most antidepressant medications, they noted. They suggest light exposure could be used to hasten antidepressant response.

Injured athletes simultaneously may experience diminished feelings of competence and self-worth and undergo an abrupt decrement in light exposure due to reduction in outdoor training. Postolache and Oren recommended that sidelined athletes continue to get bright-light exposure, either natural or artificial.

Chapter 35

Does Sleep Deprivation Lead To Weight Gain?

Researchers at the University of Chicago have found that partial sleep deprivation alters the circulating levels of the hormones that regulate hunger, causing an increase in appetite and a preference for calorie-dense, high-carbohydrate foods. The study, published in the 7 Dec. 2004 issue of the *Annals of Internal Medicine*, provides a mechanism linking sleep loss to the epidemic of obesity.

Research subjects who slept only four hours a night for two nights had an 18 percent decrease in leptin, a hormone that tells the brain there is no need for more food, and a 28 percent increase in ghrelin, a hormone that triggers hunger.

The study volunteers, all healthy young men, reported a 24 percent increase in appetite, with a surge in desire for sweets, such as candy and cookies, salty foods such as chips and nuts, and starchy foods such as bread and pasta.

"This is the first study to show that sleep is a major regulator of these two hormones and to correlate the extent of the hormonal changes with the magnitude of the hunger change," said Eve Van Cauter, PhD, professor of medicine at the University of Chicago. "It provides biochemical evidence connecting the trend toward chronic sleep curtailment to obesity and its consequences, including metabolic syndrome and diabetes."

About This Chapter: "Sleep Loss Boosts Appetite, May Encourage Weight Gain," University of Chicago Medical Center Office of Public Affairs, December 6, 2004. Reprinted with permission.

In the last 40 years, American adults have cut their average sleep time by nearly two hours. In 1960, U.S. adults slept an average of 8.5 hours a night. By 2002, that had fallen to less than seven hours a night. Over the same period, the proportion of young adults sleeping less than seven hours increased from 15.6 percent to 37.1 percent. Now, only 23.5 percent, or less than one out of four young adults, sleeps at least eight hours a night.

As sleep time fell, average weights rose. In 1960 only one out of four adults was overweight and about one out of nine was considered obese, with a body mass index of 30 or more. Now two out of three adults is overweight and nearly one out of three is obese.

Whether and how these two trends are connected, however, is unclear. Sleep-deprived rats eat more than those allowed normal sleep. Several epidemiologic studies showed that people who sleep less are more likely to be overweight. One recent study found that those who reported less than four hours of sleep a night were 73 percent more likely to be obese.

♣ It's A Fact!!

Modern scientific study of sleep began at the University of Chicago in 1953 with the discovery of rapid eye movement (REM) sleep and subsequent studies that described the multiple stages of sleep. For many years, research on the consequences of sleep deprivation focused on the brain. Since 1999, however, the Van Cauter laboratory has published a series of studies describing the metabolic and hormonal consequences of chronic partial sleep loss—which is now common. Such studies include:

- A 1999 study showing that a significant sleep debt could trigger metabolic and endocrine changes that mimic many of the hallmarks of aging.

- A 2000 paper that mapped out the stages of age-related sleep deterioration and showed how changes in sleep were mirrored by changes in hormone secretion, which in turn reduced sleep quality.

- A 2001 study demonstrating that inadequate sleep could foster insulin-resistance, a risk factor for Type 2 diabetes.

- A 2002 study showed that sleep deprivation could slow the response to vaccination, suggesting that sleep loss could reduce the ability to fight off an infection.

By providing the first data on the relationship between sleep and the hormones that regulate hunger, this study helps to confirm and begins to explain the connection.

Van Cauter and colleagues studied 12 healthy male volunteers in their early 20s to see how sleep loss affected the hormones that control appetite. Theses hormones—ghrelin and leptin, both discovered in the last 10 years—represent the 'yin-yang' of appetite regulation. Ghrelin, made by the stomach, connotes hunger. Leptin, produced by fat cells, connotes satiety, telling the brain when we have eaten enough.

Van Cauter's team measured circulating levels of leptin and ghrelin before the study, after two nights of only four hours in bed (average sleep time 3 hours and 53 minutes) and after two nights of ten hours in bed (sleep time 9 hours and 8 minutes). They used questionnaires to assess hunger and the desire for different food types.

"We were particularly interested in the ratio of the two hormones," said Van Cauter, "the balance between ghrelin and leptin."

After a night with four hours of sleep, the ration of ghrelin to leptin increased by 71 percent compared to a night with ten hours in bed.

As hunger increased, food choices changed. After two nights of curtailed sleep the volunteers found foods such as candy, cookies, and cake far more appealing. Desire for fruit, vegetables, or dairy products increased much less.

"We don't yet know why food choice would shift," Van Cauter said. "Since the brain is fueled by glucose, we suspect it seeks simple carbohydrates when distressed by lack of sleep." At the same time, the added difficulty of making decisions while sleepy may weaken the motivation to select more nutritious foods, making it harder to push away the doughnuts in favor of a low-fat yoghurt.

"Our modern industrial society seems to have forgotten the importance of sleep," Van Cauter said. "We are all under pressure to perform, in school, at work, in social, and professional settings, and tempted by multiple diversions.

There is a sense that you can pack in more of life by skimping on sleep. But we are finding that people tend to replace reduced sleep with added calories, and that's not a healthy trade."

The National Institutes of Health, the European Sleep Research Society, the Belgian Fonds de la Recherche Scientifique Medicale, the University of Chicago Diabetes Research and Training Grant and the University of Chicago Clinical Research Center funded this study. Authors include Esra Tasali and Plamen Penev of the University of Chicago and Karine Spiegel of the Universite Libre de Bruxelles, Belgium.

Chapter 36

Drowsy Driving: A Potentially Deadly Result Of Sleep Deprivation

The National Highway Traffic Safety Administration (NHTSA) conservatively estimates that 100,000 police-reported crashes are the direct result of driver fatigue each year, resulting in an estimated 1,500 deaths, 71,000 injuries, and $12.5 billion in monetary losses.

Definitions of drowsy driving generally involve varying uses and definitions of fatigue, sleepiness, and exhaustion. For the purpose of the discussion at hand, drowsy driving is simply driving in a physical state in which the driver's alertness is appreciably lower than it would be if the driver were "well rested" and "fully awake."

How serious of a problem is drowsy driving?

On the national level, the National Highway Traffic Safety Administration (NHTSA) conservatively estimates that 100,000 police-reported crashes are the direct result of driver fatigue each year, resulting in an estimated 1,500 deaths, 71,000 injuries, and $12.5 billion in monetary losses. However, it is very difficult to determine when fatigue causes or contributes to a traffic crash, and many experts believe these statistics understate the magnitude of the problem.

About This Chapter: "Frequently Asked Questions: Drowsy Driving," © 2005 AAA Foundation for Traffic Safety. Reprinted with permission.

On the individual level, driving while tired is very dangerous, because a driver who falls asleep may crash head-on into another vehicle, a tree, or a wall, at full driving speed, without making any attempt to avoid the crash by steering or braking.

The inability of a sleeping driver to try to avoid crashing makes this type of crash especially severe. Some studies have found people's cognitive-psychomotor abilities to be as impaired after 24 hours without sleep as with a blood alcohol content (BAC) of 0.10%, which is higher than the legal limit for driving while intoxicated (DWI) conviction in all U.S. states.

What are the warning signs of drowsy driving?

Some warnings signs you may experience that signify drowsiness while driving are:

- The inability to recall the last few miles traveled,

- Having disconnected or wandering thoughts,

- Having difficulty focusing or keeping your eyes open,

- Feeling as though your head is very heavy,

- Drifting out of your driving lane, perhaps driving on the rumble strips,

- Yawning repeatedly,

- Accidentally tailgating other vehicles,

- Missing traffic signs.

♣ **It's A Fact!!**

Drowsy drivers sometimes drive so poorly that they might appear to be drunk. In a survey of police officers conducted by the AAA Foundation for Traffic Safety, nearly 90 percent of responding officers had at least once pulled over a driver who they expected to find intoxicated, but turned out to be sleepy (and not intoxicated).

Source: © 2005 AAA Foundation for Traffic Safety.

What are the specific at-risk groups affected by drowsy driving?

The specific at-risk group for drowsy-driving-related crashes comprises people who drive after having not slept enough, qualitatively or quantitatively. If you're tired and you're driving, you are at risk. In general, individuals who are "most at-risk for being at-risk" of drowsy driving include:

Young People: Sleep-related crashes are most common in young people, especially those who tend to stay up late, sleep too little, and drive at night— a dangerous combination. A study by the National Highway Traffic Safety Administration and the State of New York found that young drivers are more than 4 times more likely to have sleep-related crashes than are drivers over age 30.

Shift Workers And People With Long Work Hours: Shift workers and people who work long hours are at high risk of being involved in a sleep-related crash. The human body never fully adjusts to shift work, according to the National Sleep Foundation. The body's sleep and wake cycles are dictated by light and dark cycles, and generally will lead one to feel sleepy between midnight and 6 A.M. For more information, see the National Sleep Foundation's Sleep Strategies for Shift Workers available on their website at http://www.sleepfoundation.org.

People With Undiagnosed Or Untreated Sleep Disorders: Approximately 40 million people are believed to have some kind of sleep disorder. Many different sleep disorders result in excessive daytime sleepiness, placing this group at high risk for sleep-related crashes. Common sleep disorders that often go unnoticed or undiagnosed include sleep apnea, narcolepsy, and restless leg syndrome. You can learn more about these and other sleep disorders by visiting the National Sleep Foundation website at http://www.sleep foundation.org.

Business Travelers: Business travelers struggle with jet lag, a common sleep disorder that causes sleepiness and negatively affects alertness. "Jet lag" as well as long work hours put these weary travelers at increased risk for sleep-related crashes.

Finally, it is important to realize that although these specific groups of people are statistically most likely to be involved in drowsy driving crashes, one who does not fall into any of these groups is by no means "immune" to drowsy driving. "Average drivers" who don't happen to be under age 30, working the night shift, traveling for business, or suffering from sleep apnea are still at risk if they drive while fatigued.

Do people realize how dangerous it is to drive while drowsy?

According to AAA Foundation for Traffic Safety research, the public perceives drowsy driving to be an important cause of motor vehicle crashes. Three out of four non-crash-involved drivers, and four out of five of those in recent crashes, said that driver drowsiness was "very important" in causing crashes. These results place drowsy driving as being less of a contributor to crashes in the public's view than alcohol, but more important than poor weather conditions, speeding, or driver inexperience. Drowsy driving and aggressive driving, which have both received fairly widespread media attention, were rated about the same.

What can be done in advance to avoid drowsy driving altogether?

Get A Good Night's Sleep: The amount needed varies from individual to individual, but sleep experts recommend between 7–9 hours of sleep per night.

Plan To Drive Long Trips With A Companion: Passengers can help look for early warning signs of fatigue, and switching drivers may be helpful. Passengers should stay awake and monitor the driver's condition.

✔ **Quick Tip**
Tips To Avoid Drowsy Driving

• Be well rested before hitting the road. Keep in mind that if you skimp on sleep for several nights in a row, it might take more than one night of good sleep to be well rested and alert.

• Avoid driving between midnight and 7 A.M. This period of time is when we are naturally the most sleepy.

• Don't drive alone. A companion who's awake and can keep you engaged in conversation may help you stay awake.

• Schedule frequent breaks on long road trips.

• Don't drink alcohol!

• Don't count on caffeine. Although drinking a cola or coffee might help keep you awake for a short time, it won't overcome excessive sleepiness.

Source: Excerpted from "In Brief: Your Guide to Healthy Sleep," National Heart, Lung, and Blood Institute, April 2006.

Take Regular Breaks: Schedule regular stops—every 100 miles or two hours, even if you don't feel tired, and more often if you feel like you need it.

Avoid Alcohol And Medications: If medications warn that they cause or may cause drowsiness, avoid taking them before driving. If you must take certain prescription medications that cause drowsiness, don't drive immediately after taking them.

Teens should never consume alcohol—especially before driving because it interacts with fatigue, and increases sleepiness. If you are already tired, even a small quantity of alcohol may exacerbate your sleepiness and increase your risk of crashing, even if your BAC is well below the legal limit for a DWI conviction.

Consult Your Physician Or A Local Sleep Disorders Center: If you suffer frequent daytime sleepiness, experience difficulty sleeping at night, and/or snore loudly on a regular basis, consult your physician or local sleep disorders center for a diagnosis and treatment.

For more information about sleep, sleep disorders, and the effects of sleeping too little, visit the National Sleep Foundation website at http://www.sleep foundation.org.

♣ **It's A Fact!!**

True or False? More people doze off at the wheel of a car in the early morning or midafternoon than in the evening.

True. Our bodies are programmed by our biological clock to experience two natural periods of sleepiness during the 24-hour day, regardless of the amount of sleep we've had in the previous 24 hours. The primary period is between about midnight and 7:00 A.M. A second period of less intense sleepiness is in the midafternoon, between about 1:00 and 3:00. This means that we are more at risk of falling asleep at the wheel at these times than in the evening—especially if we haven't been getting enough sleep.

Source: Excerpted from "Test Your Sleep IQ," National Heart, Lung, and Blood Institute, 2006.

When are drowsy driving crashes most likely to occur?

As intuition dictates and data confirms, most sleep crashes occur in the "middle of the night," during the early morning hours. Less obviously, though, there is also a peak in sleep-related crashes in the mid-afternoon. Our natural circadian rhythms dictate that we will be most sleepy during the middle of our nighttime sleep period, and again about 12 hours later, between 2 P.M. and 4 P.M., and various studies show a peak in crashes believed to be related to sleep somewhere between 2 P.M. and 6 P.M.

What if I'm already driving and I start to feel tired? What should I do?

Take a nap. Naps are beneficial when experiencing drowsiness. Find a safe place (i.e., not the shoulder of the highway) where you can stop, park your car, and sleep for 15 to 20 minutes. A nap longer than 20 minutes can make you groggy for at least 15 minutes after awakening.

If you are planning a long trip, or routinely drive for long durations, identify safe places to stop and nap. If you only have a short distance remaining (e.g., an hour or so of driving), the nap might be enough to revive you. If you still have several hours of driving planned, and you're already feeling tired, it would probably be best to find a bed for the night, get a full night's sleep, and then resume driving.

♣ It's A Fact!!
True or False? Opening the car window or turning the radio up will keep the drowsy driver awake.

False. Opening the car window or turning the radio up may arouse a drowsy driver briefly, but this won't keep that person alert behind the wheel. Even mild drowsiness is enough to reduce concentration and reaction time. The sleep-deprived driver may nod off for a couple of seconds at a time without even knowing it—enough time to kill himself or someone else. It has been estimated that drowsy driving may account for an average of 56,000 reported accidents each year—claiming over 1,500 lives.

Source: Excerpted from "Test Your Sleep IQ," National Heart, Lung, and Blood Institute, 2006.

What about coffee? Won't that keep me awake?

Not necessarily. The "perk" that comes from drinking a cup of coffee may take a half hour or so to "kick in," is relatively short in duration, and will be less effective for those who regularly consume caffeine (i.e., most people). If you're very sleepy, and rely on caffeine to allow you to continue driving, you are likely to experience "microsleeps," in which you doze off for four or five seconds, which doesn't sound like long, but is still plenty of time to drive off of the road or over the centerline and crash.

☞ **Remember!!**

If you are short on sleep, stay out of the driver's seat!

Source: Excerpted from "In Brief: Your Guide to Healthy Sleep," National Heart, Lung, and Blood Institute, April 2006.

Should I open the window or turn up the radio to fight fatigue on the road?

No. Some of these tricks may help you to feel more alert for an instant; however, they are not effective ways to maintain an acceptable level of alertness for long enough to drive anywhere. Even with the window rolled all the way down and radio cranked up, if you're sleepy, you're still an unnecessarily great hazard to yourself and to everybody else on the road. If you're sleepy enough that you're seeking special measures to stay awake, you should have stopped driving already. Look for a safe and secure place, park the car, and take a nap.

Are there any devices I can buy that will keep me awake while I'm driving?

There are a few devices on the market, some of which are worn on your body or placed in your car, that are advertised to keep drowsy drivers awake; however, to our knowledge, none of them have been scientifically validated yet. The only driver warning mechanism that has been validated to date is the shoulder rumblestrip, which produces noise and mechanical vibration if your vehicle drives on it. If you start driving onto the rumblestrip, this is an indication that you are too tired to drive safely. You should not rely on the rumblestrip to alert you every time you begin to doze off and drive off course— rumblestrips won't prevent you from crashing into other cars.

Part Five

Sleep Research

Chapter 37

America's Sleepy Teens: A Look At The Numbers

It's not just growth spurts, new hairdos, and fashion crazes that mark the onset of adolescence. Sleep experts say that changing sleep patterns are markers for adolescence, too. Though teens need more sleep than adults, they are more likely to feel wide awake until late at night and can more naturally sleep later into the morning. Pit this pattern against early school schedules, the desire to load up on courses or activities and a 24/7 world of electronic options and you have a recipe for...

America's Sleepy Teens

The National Sleep Foundation's (NSF) 2006 Sleep in America poll conducted during fall 2005 randomly surveyed 1,602 households across the U.S. The poll, fashioned by experts on adolescent sleep, asked questions of one family member between the ages of 11 and 17 and one parent or guardian in the same household in order to compare their responses.

The findings provide a first-time data-based portrait of America's adolescents and how they sleep.

About This Chapter: From "2006 Sleep in America Poll," National Sleep Foundation (http://www.sleepfoundation.org), © 2006; reprinted with permission.

Lauren's Cram-Packed Day: When sixteen year-old Lauren gets home from a full day of school, cheerleading practice, and a quick bite to eat, she's full of energy and life. After IM'ing on her computer, talking on the phone, and working on some homework, she still feels wired and is reluctant to go to sleep. Because Lauren's parents are used to seeing their daughter come to life at night, they often have a hard time convincing her to go bed; they can't really imagine that she is sleep deprived. Yet what they often don't notice is that Lauren has trouble waking up in the morning, can't get going until she's had a cup of coffee, is groggy when she heads off to school, yawns throughout the morning and has difficulty paying attention in many of her classes. Because she manages to stay afloat in school, participates in extracurricular activities, and makes time for friends, Lauren is perceived to be an "average" teenager with a busy schedule and little time for sleep. No one realizes that there are two sides to Lauren's day and personality—at night she's an energetic teenager who makes time for family and friends; during the day she's often an irritable, sleepy teen who is struggling to balance her responsibilities.

Like many other adolescents and their parents surveyed in NSF's 2006 Sleep in America poll, Lauren and her family have been fooled by what Jodi Mindell, associate director of the Sleep Disorders Center at the Children's Hospital of Philadelphia, calls the "trick of nature." According to Mindell, adolescents' circadian rhythms change when they hit adolescence—their brains and bodies are geared to stay awake later and sleep in later, but their school schedules don't permit this kind of lifestyle. Parents often observe an alert, active teen at night without realizing that many of the signs of sleep deprivation regularly show themselves in the morning. To compound this problem, many parents and teens don't realize that sleep experts recommend that adolescents get 8.5 to 9.25 hours of sleep every night as a minimum. To this mix of circadian rhythms and additional sleep needs, add in a busy social life, extracurricular activities, sports and a job and the result is that America's teenagers are constantly fighting against their brains' and bodies' natural tendencies.

Like Lauren, the majority of NSF poll respondents are not getting the sleep they need, and the consequences are catching up with them in all areas of their lives. For instance, in response to the poll, many teens said they often arrive late for school, fall asleep in class, and are too tired to exercise. As they deal with numerous social and academic pressures, the lives of adolescents only become busier as they get older, while sufficient sleep becomes a distant memory for many.

Coping With Sleep Deprivation

> ### ♣ It's A Fact!!
>
> For professionals in the sleep field, the National Sleep Foundation's (NSF) poll results are disturbing—trends indicate that not only are adolescents shortchanging themselves when it comes to getting enough sleep, but adolescents' parents may be in the dark about the "sleep debt" their children may be accumulating. "It is difficult for families to plan for sufficient sleep nowadays," says Mary Carskadon, a sleep researcher at Brown University and chair of the National Sleep Foundation (NSF) poll taskforce. "So many 'essential' activities get jammed into every day."

According To The Poll: Only 20% of adolescents report that they get an optimal nine hours of sleep on school nights and nearly half say they actually sleep less than eight hours on school nights.

The NSF poll found that many teens try to "cut corners" when it comes to staying alert during the day, trying to fend off sleepiness rather than getting the sleep they need. These coping behaviors are increasingly apparent with each year of adolescence; older teens (12th graders) report getting just 6.9 hours of sleep on average.

Results of NSF's 2006 Sleep in America poll show that many teens have adopted unhealthy behaviors including:

- Napping: 38% of surveyed high school students took at least two naps per week in the two weeks preceding their poll interview.

- Sleeping late on weekends: Most adolescents are sleeping between 1.2 and 1.9 hours longer on non-school nights.

- Frequently consuming caffeinated beverages and foods: 31% of those surveyed drink two or more caffeinated beverages a day.

- Giving up on exercise: More than a quarter (28%) of adolescents say they felt too tired or sleepy to exercise.

- Driving drowsy: More than half (51%) who drive say they've driven while drowsy during the past year.

While teens and many adults often rely on these strategies as coping mechanisms to make it through the day, these habits are often signs of sleep deprivation and may intensify difficulty sleeping, decrease performance in school, work and activities, and can even pose danger to themselves and others.

Effects Of Sleep Deprivation On Mood

According To The Poll: More than half (55%) of adolescents with the best mood score can say "I had a good night's sleep" every night or almost every night vs. only 20% of those with the worst mood score.

In the NSF poll, every adolescent was asked five questions derived from a recognized mental health questionnaire to gauge the outlook and mood of each respondent. The results of the poll indicated that the effects of sleep deprivation can also impact adolescents' mood, behavior and attitude. While some parents might think "all teens are moody," or it is natural for teens to act irritable and irrational, in fact, lack of sleep can cause teens to act out and succumb to feelings of anxiety, depression, and hopelessness.

The NSF poll showed that among those adolescents with the best and worst mood scores there was little difference for factors like body mass index, time spent exercising each week, employment, use of caffeine, or grades, but those with the worst mood scores were more than twice as likely to have trouble falling asleep than those with the best scores (51% vs. 18%) and were about three times as likely to say they "felt too tired during the day" (59% vs. 19%). An upshot of these findings from the NSF poll: with further research, such sleep-related factors may be used to more quickly identify and help children with mood disorders. Improving their sleep may be the first step in stemming greater mental health problems.

☞ Remember!!
"Insufficient sleep not only results in difficulty with focus, attention, and concentration making it difficult to excel in school but also leads to irritability and mood disorder," says Helene Emsellem, medical director at the Center for Sleep and Wake Disorders in Chevy Chase, Maryland.

School

According To The Poll: More than a quarter (28%) of high school students report that they fell asleep in school at least once a week in the past two weeks; 14% say they arrived late or missed school because they overslept.

The poll found that adolescents' average school day begins around 6:30 A.M. In fact, 52% of American high school students start school before 8 A.M. and on average they leave the house by 7:10 A.M. To top off early start times, busy school days and afternoon and early evening activities, 55% of high school students don't go to bed until after 11 P.M. on school nights, likely resulting from their natural sleep phase delay as well as their busy routine.

> ## ♣ It's A Fact!!
>
> The place where sleep problems are most likely to present themselves is also the place where parents may not know that sleep problems occur and where everyone is concerned about performance—school. Many teachers and parents who witness an adolescent falling asleep in class, arriving late to school, or underperforming each semester may blame it on the adolescent's "laziness", boredom, or apathy towards school. Yet results of the National Sleep Foundation (NSF)'s 2006 Sleep in America poll indicate that lack of sleep or poor sleep quality may be a reason for such problems.

The NSF poll also found that students who get sufficient sleep perform better in school, with 34% reporting better grades than those who didn't get the minimum recommended sleep. "Many parents (and teens) think that teens have to stay up late to study and be successful," says Judith Owens, director of the pediatric sleep disorders clinic at Hasbro Children's Hospital in Providence, Rhode Island. "The poll results support other studies which show the opposite is true; A and B students report going to bed earlier and getting more sleep than students with poorer grades."

Sleep Environment

According To The Poll: 57% of 9th-12th graders have cell phones in their bedroom, while only 21% of 6th graders do.

While sleep professionals recommend that all individuals should enjoy relaxing activities before bed, the best thing to do in the bedroom is sleep. High-tech "sleep stealers" such as televisions, computers, cell phones, and MP3 players not only cut into sleep time, but they often make their user feel active and alert when they're used near bedtime and/or in the bedroom. For many adolescents, technology is encroaching on a good night's sleep. More things are competing for their time, and in a high-tech, 24/7 world, sending instant messages to friends, talking on the phone, or surfing the internet can be inviting outlets for teens when the day has been hectic and filled with stressors.

The poll confirms that whether or not adolescents are choosing gadgets over sleep, they certainly have the opportunity to do so: 90% of adolescents have MP3 players or radios in their bedrooms and 57% have TVs in their rooms. Plus, how "wired" an adolescent's bedroom is may be linked with age—the poll indicates that the number of "sleep stealers" increases as adolescents grow older.

Some other common "sleep stealers" among adolescents include internet access in the bedroom (21% of adolescents) and video games or cell phones in the bedroom (43% and 42% respectively).

The poll shows that the hour before bedtime is also filled with numerous alerting activities— four in ten adolescents went on the internet or talked on the phone within an hour before going to bed. Activities such as playing video games, watching television, and exercising in the hour before bedtime are more common for males than females, but the poll shows that the majority of all adolescents seem to have a stimulating activity of

✔ Quick Tip
How Teens Can Avoid The Trick Of Nature

- Instead of waiting to see if you "crash" at night, look for signs of sleepiness during the day, especially in the morning.

- Ask yourself and answer honestly: "How often would you say you get a good night's sleep?"

- Pay attention to your caffeine consumption, napping, and mood.

- Establish consistent sleep and wake schedules.

- Learn about the importance of sleep.

- Keep "sleep stealers" out of your bedroom—keep the TV and computer in a different room instead.

choice before bedtime, rather than an activity conducive to sleep. Dr. Owens recommends that parents should "sometimes set limits on things like the amount of TV teens watch, the number of caffeinated beverages they drink, the hours during which they are allowed to call their friends, the number of extracurricular activities that they participate in, and the hours that they work at after-school jobs" in order to help their children make choices when an endless amount of day and nighttime activities present themselves.

The Role Of Parents

According To The Poll: Only 7% of caregivers think their adolescent may have a sleep problem, but 16% of adolescents report thinking they have or may have one. Yet, 31% of those adolescents who think they may have a sleep problem have not told anyone about it.

What is causing such a drastic disparity between caregivers' perceptions and their children's actions?

One explanation might be that, as a society, Americans often put sleep on the backburner. The 2005 Sleep in America poll showed that on average, American adults are only getting 6.9 hours of sleep a night, less than sleep professionals' recommended 7–9 hours. Sleep-deprived adults may be so accustomed to their own tired state that they may not recognize sleep problems in their children. With an increasing dependency on caffeinated beverages to get through the day, both adolescents and adults may be "masking" their sleep debt.

The "two-sided" behavior of teens may also fool parents into believing that their children are well-rested. Because the circadian rhythms of adolescents compel them to go to bed later and arise later, parents are likely to mistakenly label their teens' obstinacy about bedtime as "typical teenage behavior" rather than a facet of their biology. "This is the 'trick of nature' that Dr. Mindell is referring to," says NSF CEO Richard Gelula. "The adolescent doesn't necessarily feel or appear sleepy at night when other family members do and remains active later, but the scheduled wake-up time occurs too early, resulting in sleep deprivation and daytime sleepiness as well as impaired cognitive abilities, mood and physical performance."

Parents may also not realize that signs of sleep deprivation commonly appear in the morning, rather than at night. They may expect that it is "normal" to be sleepy for the first hour after waking up, or that their teen is "bored" or apathetic about school which causes them to fall asleep in class. In fact, these signs, along with others such as irritability and dependency on caffeine, indicate that teens may be suffering from sleep deprivation and aren't the happy-go-lucky people they appear to be when they get a burst of energy in the evening.

Results And Making Changes

NSF's 2006 Sleep in America poll shows that America's adolescents are caught up in a complex juggling act. As they mature, teenagers are increasingly challenged to take responsibility for difficult choices about their schedules and daily habits. Yet as set bedtimes fade away, sleep is often put at the bottom of the to-do list.

Helping teens navigate the choices of the 24/7 world seems more of a priority now than ever. Teens at the very least need exposure to a health education that includes a focus on sleep, how to get it and how to recognize and respond constructively to sleep problems. They also need to be able to communicate about sleep with their parents or guardians and with their primary care doctor. At the community level, everyone is responsible for seeing that schedules affecting teens' lives are developed in a realistic way that is informed by sleep biology and a balanced perspective on teen needs.

"If parents and teens know what good sleep entails and the benefits of making and sticking to a plan that supports good sleep, then they might need to do a better job making choices about what truly are the 'essential' activities," says Dr. Carskadon. "The earlier parents can start helping their children with good sleep habits, the easier it will be to sustain them through the teen years."

Chapter 38

A Good Night's Sleep May Be Key To Effective Learning

Robert Stickgold, PhD, wants you to know that your mother was right—you really should be getting more sleep.

Stickgold, a professor of psychiatry at Harvard Medical School, believes that sleep allows us to process, consolidate, and retain new memories and skills. In his lab, he investigates sleep's effects on students who learn new tasks, such as complex finger-tapping sequences. He's found that depriving the students of a night's sleep afterward significantly cuts back on how well they remember the new skill as much as three days later.

The idea that people need sleep to consolidate memories has waxed and waned in popularity since psychologists John Jenkins and Karl Dallenbach first proposed that sleep benefits memory more than 80 years ago. In the last 10 years, evidence from memory studies in humans and rats, as well as research on the cellular and molecular workings of the brain, have provided increasing evidence for the link.

Now, researchers are investigating which sorts of memories might be consolidated during sleep and which stages of sleep are important—after all, sleep is not a monolithic entity but is divided into stages that cycle back and forth, from the most active (rapid eye movement, or REM) to the least active (slow wave sleep).

Still, the theory remains controversial. And the details remain elusive—partially because scientists don't entirely understand how the brain retains memories at all. Without that knowledge, it's difficult to be certain of how—or even if—sleep contributes to the process.

"It would have been nice if the memory researchers had worked everything out," says Stickgold, "but it turns out we may be able to help them some."

An Old Idea, New Interest

Several researchers studied sleep and memory in the 1960s and 70s, but the number of studies in the area tapered off during the 1980s. The most recent spate of interest in memory and learning took off in 1994, after an influential paper published in *Science* (Vol. 265, No. 5,172, pages 679–682) helped revive the field, according to Stickgold.

In that study, neuroscientist Avi Karni, MD, PhD, trained participants to report whether they'd seen horizontal or vertical lines appear over a background pattern on a computer screen while they focused elsewhere on the screen. Most participants took about 100 milliseconds to identify the lines' orientation. But when the participants returned the next day after a normal night's sleep, they were able to do the task about 15 milliseconds faster—and the improvement lasted for a year. When researchers kept the participants in the lab overnight and woke them every time they fell into REM sleep, they didn't improve at all.

Stickgold and others have followed up on this study, examining such questions as whether sleep stages other than REM may be involved. In a 2000 study, for example, Stickgold found that participants' improvement on the line-identifying task depended on how much slow wave sleep they got during the first quarter of the night and how much REM sleep they got during the last quarter of the night.

"The more you sleep, the more improvement you show—it's really a nice linear relationship," Stickgold says.

♣ It's A Fact!!

With the busy schedules teens keep, who can afford inefficient studying re-reading the same page while being too tired to focus, nodding off in class, or staying up late to study, only to be unable to recall the information the next day?

It can be tempting for teens to sacrifice sleep to squeeze studying and other activities into an already full day. But less sleep does not equal more time. Research shows that sleep deprivation in teens—even if they are consistently getting just a few hours less than they need each night—can impair their ability to learn and hurt their overall performance.

Research shows that sleep deprivation impairs:

• Ability to pay attention

• Verbal creativity and effective communication

• Abstract thinking

• Creative problem-solving and innovation

• Mental sharpness (the sleep-deprived person is more vulnerable to misleading remarks and has more difficulty with complex, ambiguous material)

• Decision-making involving the unexpected

• Adaptive learning that involves retrieving knowledge from long-term memory, adding to that knowledge, and using it to solve problems

• Overall mood and motivation

Studies also show that when learning certain types of tasks, those who get a good night's sleep afterward perform better when tested the next day than those who get insufficient sleep. In fact, researchers have found that after a person learns new information, there is activity in the same area of the brain during sleep, and there is improvement in memory performance when the person is tested the next day. So getting a good night's sleep after learning something new is a crucial step in organizing new information and strengthening recent memories.

Source: "From ZZZ's to A's: Sleep and Learning," © 2007 National Sleep Foundation (www.sleepfoundation.org). All rights reserved. Reprinted with permission.

In a follow-up study, he showed that sleep deprivation the night after training blocked improvement on the task even after participants had two nights of normal sleep to recover.

In another study, Stickgold taught participants to tap out a number sequence on a keyboard. Students improved their speed on the task with practice for a few minutes, but then quickly reached a peak performance level. A control group of students who were tested 12 hours later on the same day showed no more improvement on the task, but those who went home and slept overnight improved 20 percent by the next day, although they had not practiced any more.

Of course, these studies tested procedural rather than declarative memory. Procedural memories are memories for motor and perceptual skills like riding a bike or hitting a baseball—or tapping numbers on a keyboard. Declarative memories, on the other hand, are memories of facts like the capital of North Dakota or a friend's birthday.

Evidence for sleep's effect on declarative memory is much weaker than for its effect on procedural memory. In fact, few studies have shown any link between the two. Still, says Stickgold, even this distinction is less sharp than it might seem—sleep may affect "complex procedural" memories, like the ability to synthesize new information with old and develop new ideas.

In fact, a 2004 *Nature* study by German neuroscientist Jan Born, MD, of the University of Lübeck, found evidence for just that (Vol. 427, No. 6,972, pages 352–355). Born gave participants a math test that required them to use a set of complex rules to convert eight-number strings of digits into new, seven-number strings, and then to identify the last number in the new string. But there was a trick to make this task easier: the second number the participants calculated was always the same as the last number of the new string.

When the participants first took the test, none recognized the trick. After a night of sleep, though, 13 out of 22 participants caught on. Only 5 out of 22 participants who were retested after the equivalent amount of daytime wakefulness got it.

"If you're going to be tested on 72 irregular French verbs tomorrow, you might as well stay up late and cram," Stickgold says. "But if they're going to throw a curveball at you and ask you to explain the differences between the French Revolution and the Industrial Revolution, you're better off having gotten some sleep."

♣ It's A Fact!!
Don't Settle For Less!

Chronically sleep-deprived teens can become so used to the sensation of sleepiness that they "settle" for less than they are capable of in creativity, academic performance, and communication both in and out of the classroom.

Certain tasks, especially those that are rule-based, logical, or very exciting and engaging, can be less sensitive to sleep deprivation and give the misperception that a person's overall learning and performance is at its best. For example, research shows that a sleep-deprived person may be able to memorize facts but then be unable to use that information in a constructive and innovative way. A person may be able to say something logical, but be unable to come up with spontaneous ideas or handle unpredictable situations.

Source: "From ZZZ's to A's: Sleep and Learning," © 2007 National Sleep Foundation (www.sleepfoundation.org). All rights reserved. Reprinted with permission.

What's Going On Inside The Brain

Studies of human learning provide tantalizing evidence that sleep helps us retain new memories, but they don't provide information about how it does so. For that, most researchers turn to animal studies. Scientists are exploring a few lines of evidence, most of which, by necessity, approach the issue of memory obliquely. University of Pennsylvania neuroscientist Marcos Frank, PhD, for example, is studying how sleep influences brain cell plasticity—the ability to form new synapses and connections between brain cells. Researchers know that brain cell plasticity is key to creating and retaining memories, but because scientists don't know precisely where memories are stored in the brain, they can't look for "new-memory" synapses directly.

Instead, Frank is examining how sleep affects plasticity in the visual cortex of cats. He blocks the cats' vision in one eye for a few hours when the cats are young, which causes cells in the visual cortex to remodel themselves to respond less strongly to the deprived eye. In a 2001 study in *Neuron* (Vol. 30, No. 1, pages 275–287), Frank blocked cats' vision for six hours while allowing them to explore their environments in a lighted room. Then he tested the synaptic remodeling that resulted. In the next phase of the experiment, he allowed one group of cats to sleep for six hours and kept another group awake in the dark. He found that the synaptic remodeling continued for the extra six hours in the sleep group, but not in the waking group.

"We're not studying sleep and memory per se, but we are studying a model of how the brain can change its structure with experience," Frank says. "We found that sleep does seem to play a role in this plasticity and enhance changes that are already taking place."

Now, Frank and his colleagues are working to isolate the particular sleep stages—REM or non-REM—that contribute most to this plasticity.

Other researchers, meanwhile, are looking at a smaller level than cells—they're investigating genes.

Neuroscientist Sidarta Ribeiro, PhD, for example, has studied a gene called zif-268, which is related to brain plasticity. When activated, the gene activates a protein called synapsin II, which promotes the formation of new synapses. In a 1999 study, Ribeiro allowed rats to explore a new environment—thus creating new memories—and then to sleep for several hours. He found that during the REM sleep that followed, the zif-268 gene was more active in the rats' cerebral cortexes and hippocampi—the areas thought to be important for memory.

"The hippocampus is the entrance gate for memories, and then they migrate to the cortex," Ribeiro explains.

He, like Frank, is now working to sort out the contribution that slow wave sleep makes to the process as well.

The Other Side

Studies like these, and dozens of others, have convinced most sleep researchers that sleep plays an important and unique role in human memory. But a few scientists vehemently disagree with their findings. One of the most vocal detractors is psychologist and neuroscientist Robert Vertes, PhD, who studies memory at Florida Atlantic University.

One of his central arguments comes from the widespread use of antidepressants. Older antidepressants, such as monoamine oxidase inhibitors (MAOIs), completely eliminate REM sleep in users, and even the newer selective serotonin reuptake inhibitor (SSRI) antidepressants can significantly reduce REM sleep for months or years. Given the huge number of people who've taken these drugs, Vertes asks, why haven't we seen widespread reports of memory impairment?

"They'd pull these drugs off the market if people were saying 'They're making me senile,'" he says.

Supporters of the memory consolidation theory point out that it's possible that functions associated with REM sleep could migrate to other sleep stages in a person deprived of REM sleep for a long time. And, they say, just because people are not self-reporting memory problems doesn't mean that those problems aren't occurring.

"Bill Gates has been quoted saying that his programmers can program for 72 hours straight," Stickgold says. "And I say—yeah, but their product is Windows."

But Vertes and some others—including, perhaps most notably, psychologist Jerome Siegel, PhD—remain unconvinced. There are too many questions that the theory fails to answer, they say. For example, if our brains consolidate memories during REM sleep, why is it that our dreams—our only window into the brain's activity during that sleep stage—so rarely relate to anything we want to remember?

And what about new memories that a person acquires during his or her first waking hours? Where are they held during the 12 to 16 hours until that person goes back to sleep?

Remember!!

Since so much of what teens are learning is important for school, sports, and other activities, as well as for discovering the strengths and interests that can shape their lives in the short and long term, it is important to make sure teens are getting enough sleep to feel, look, and act their best!

Source: "From ZZZ's to A's: Sleep and Learning," © 2007 National Sleep Foundation (www.sleepfoundation.org). All rights reserved. Reprinted with permission.

Overall, Vertes says, he just doesn't find the memory consolidation studies convincing. "I believe that memory is online, not offline," he says.

Stickgold agrees that his critics raise points researchers need to address.

"I think every issue Siegel and Vertes raise is important," he says. "But they're not death knells for the field—they're the questions that arise as a field matures."

Further Reading

Stickgold, R. (2005). Sleep-dependent memory consolidation. *Nature*, 437(7063), 1272–1278.

Vertes, R.P. (2004). Memory consolidation in sleep: Dream or reality. *Neuron*, 44(1), 135–148.

Chapter 39

Studying The Benefits Of Delayed School Start Times

Backgrounder: Later Start Times

Adolescents today face a widespread chronic health problem: sleep deprivation. Although society often views sleep as a luxury that ambitious or active people cannot afford, research shows that getting enough sleep is a biological necessity, as important to good health as eating well or exercising. Teens are among those least likely to get enough sleep; while they need on average 9¼ hours of sleep per night for optimal performance, health and brain development, teens average fewer than 7 hours per school night by the end of high school, and most report feeling tired during the day (Wolfson & Carskadon, 1998). The roots of the problem include poor teen sleep habits that do not allow for enough hours of quality sleep; hectic schedules with after-school activities and jobs, homework hours and family obligations; and a clash between societal demands, such as early school start times, and biological changes that put most teens on a later sleep-wake clock. As a result, when it is time to wake up for school, the adolescent's body says it is still the middle of the night, and he or she has had too little sleep to feel rested and alert.

The consequences of sleep deprivation during the teenage years are particularly serious. Teens spend a great portion of each day in school; however, they are unable to maximize the learning opportunities afforded by the education system, since sleep deprivation impairs their ability to be alert, pay attention, solve problems, cope with stress and retain information. Young people who do not get enough sleep night after night carry a significant risk for fall asleep automobile crashes; emotional and behavioral problems such as irritability, depression, poor impulse control and violence; health complaints; tobacco and alcohol use; impaired cognitive function and decision-making; and lower overall performance in everything from academics to athletics.

The Biology Of Adolescent Sleep

Research shows that adolescents require at least as much sleep as they did as children, generally 8½ to 9¼ hours each night (Carskadon et al., 1980). Key changes in sleep patterns and needs during puberty can contribute to excessive sleepiness in adolescents, which can impair daytime functioning. First, daytime sleepiness can increase during adolescence, even when teens' schedules allow for optimal amounts of sleep (Carskadon, Vieri, & Acebo, 1993). Second, most adolescents undergo a sleep phase delay, which means a tendency toward later times for both falling asleep and waking up. Research shows the typical adolescent's natural time to fall asleep may be 11 P.M. or later; because of this change in their internal clocks, teens may feel wide awake at bedtime, even when they are exhausted (Wolfson & Carskadon, 1998). This leads to sleep deprivation in many teens who must wake up early for school, and thus do not get the 8½–9¼ hours of sleep that they need. It also causes irregular sleep patterns that can hurt the quality of sleep, since the weekend sleep schedule often ends up being much different from the weekday schedule as teens try to catch up on lost sleep (Dahl & Carskadon, 1995).

Adolescents In Study Show Changing Sleep Patterns

Since the 1970s, there has been a growing awareness of the changes in sleep patterns as children transition to adolescence. In a study at a summer sleep camp at Stanford during the 1970s, boys and girls who enrolled at

♣ It's A Fact!!
A Look At How Changing School Start Times Can Help!

Patricia wakes up at 5:30 every morning to get ready for school, go to track practice, sit through 7 periods of classes, and drive directly to SAT tutoring and home just in time to write her term paper. At some point she also gulps down a couple of sodas and inhales a bag of chips while catching up with her girl-friends and trying to find a date to homecoming. When her mother comes up the stairs at 11 P.M. to tell Patricia to go to sleep, she finds her daughter IM'ing with friends, watching television, and doodling in her notepad. Patricia says she is not that sleepy. Despite the fact that she has to wake up at 5:30 A.M. again tomorrow, she feels wide awake, and finds plenty of things to do.

The following Saturday morning Patricia's mother lets her daughter sleep in until noon. She figures that her overworked child could use the extra time in bed. That night, when Patricia's mom is fast asleep, Patricia cannot sleep and stays up until 2 A.M. It will not be easy to wake up at 8 A.M. Sunday morning for her charity car wash.

Patricia does manage to get up in time for the car wash, drinking a huge cup of coffee to help her through the day. When she returns home at 4 P.M. she crashes in the living room until dinner. Now that she has become accustomed to going to sleep and sleeping later or napping, you can bet that she isn't sleepy when the rest of her family turns in for the night. The cycle of sleepiness for the week is off to a bad start, because Patricia knows she has math team before school the next day.

Patricia, like many in her age group, is affected by psychosocial and biologi-cal pressures to stay up and rise later. Studies show that the typical high school student's natural time to fall asleep is often around 11:00 P.M. Research shows that adolescents require at least as much sleep as they did as children, generally 9 to 9½ hours each night. National Sleep Foundation's (NSF) 2004 *Sleep in America* poll found that the situation may be even worse: parents said that more than three-fourths of teens 13–18 go to bed 11:00 P.M. or later on school nights. Yet most high schools in the U.S. start by 7:30 A.M. and with busing, teens are getting up as early as 6 A.M., leaving most with a big sleep debt.

10–12 years of age were monitored every year for 5–6 years. While researchers had thought older children would need less sleep during the 10 hour nocturnal window they were given, from 10 P.M. to 8 A.M., they found that regardless of age, the children all slept about 9¼ of the 10 hours. As they progressed through adolescence, participants continued to get the same amount of sleep, but they no longer woke spontaneously before the end of the sleep window at 8 A.M. (Carskadon et al., 1979). In addition, when the Multiple Sleep Latency Test (MSLT)—given at designated periods throughout the day to determine the speed of falling asleep, to measure sleepiness—was given to the adolescents, they showed more alertness at 8 P.M. than earlier in the day, and even greater alertness at 10 P.M. Also, at mid-puberty, adolescents became sleepier in the middle of the day. According to the tests, more mature adolescents showed signs of reduced alertness during the day even though they slept an equivalent amount at night (Carskadon et al., 1980).

Changes In Melatonin

Another experiment, conducted by Dr. Mary A. Carskadon of Brown University, found that more mature adolescents had later circadian rhythm timing, based on melatonin secretions in saliva samples. This finding shows that melatonin secretion occurs at a later time in adolescents as they mature;

♣ It's A Fact!!

"Given that the primary focus of education is to maximize human potential, then a new task before us is to ensure that the conditions in which learning takes place address the very biology of our learners," says Mary A. Carskadon, PhD, Director of E.P. Bradley Hospital Research Laboratory and professor in Department of Psychiatry and Human Behavior at Brown University School of Medicine.

Source: "Backgrounder: Research, Advocacy, Later Start Times," © 2007 National Sleep Foundation.

thus, it is difficult for them to go to sleep earlier at night. The melatonin secretion also turns off later in the morning, which makes it harder to wake up early (Carskadon et al., 1998).

Another important finding from many studies is that the circadian timing system can be reset if light exposure is carefully controlled (Carskadon et al., 1997). In studies where adolescents are paid to keep a specific sleep schedule and wear eyeshades to exclude light during evening hours, measurements of melatonin secretion show that the rhythm had moved significantly toward a designated time. This means that with time, effort, and money, researchers can get adolescents to reset their clocks. This approach, however, is not necessarily realistic for teens who have full and busy lives. Nevertheless, the interaction of light exposure and sleep timing is important to keep in mind.

A Widespread And High-Impact Part Of Teens' Lives

Findings of the tendency for adolescent sleep patterns to be delayed have been reported not only in North America, but also in South America, Asia, Australia and Europe (Andrade & Menna Barreto, 2002; Carskadon & Acebo, 1997; Ishihara, Honma & Miyake, 1990; Bearpark & Michie, 1987; Strauch & Meier, 1988; LeBourgeois et al., 2005; Thorleifsdottir et al., 2002). The diversity of such research supports the view that intrinsic developmental changes play a role in delayed sleep patterns in adolescents. This biological shift sets the stage for other social and environmental conditions that make it easier for these adolescents to stay awake at night and wake up sleep deprived. The effects of changing sleep patterns are compounded by the demands older students face in academics, extracurricular activities, social opportunities, after-school jobs, and other obligations.

The School Start Time Issue

Adolescent sleep deprivation is largely driven by a conflict between teens' internal biological clocks and the schedules and demands of society. Therefore, it makes sense to look at school start times, which set the rhythm of the day for students, parents, teachers, and members of the community at large.

Research On School Start Times And Biology

In a project spearheaded by Dr. Mary A. Carskadon and colleagues, researchers investigated what would happen to sleep and circadian rhythms in a group of young people for whom the transition from junior high to senior high required a change in school starting time from 8:25 A.M. to 7:20 A.M. (Carskadon et al., 1998).

The 25 students completed the study at two time points, in the spring of 9th grade and autumn of 10th grade. The students kept their usual schedules, wore small activity monitors on their wrists, and kept diaries of activities and sleep schedules for two consecutive weeks. At the end, participants came to Carskadon's sleep lab for assessment of the onset phase of melatonin secretion, an overnight sleep study, and daytime testing with MSLT. The in-lab sleep schedule was fixed to each student's average school night schedule, based on data from the wrist monitors.

Carskadon and colleagues found that in the 10th grade:

- On a typical school morning, the students woke up earlier for high school, but only 25 minutes earlier instead of the 65 minutes reflected in the start time change.

- Sleep onset times did not change, and averaged about 10:40 P.M. in both 9th and 10th grade.

- The average amount of sleep on school nights fell from 7 hours 9 minutes to 6 hours 50 minutes, which is significant because the students were already accumulating a sleep deficit.

- Nearly one-half of the 10th graders showed a reversed sleep pattern on the morning MSLT. This pattern is similar to the sleep disorder narcolepsy, moving immediately into REM sleep before non-REM sleep. The 12 students who showed this pattern did not have narcolepsy, but they did have a mismatch between their school day waking times and their circadian rhythms. Indeed, at 8:30 in the morning, they fell asleep within three minutes.

- None of the students made an optimal adjustment to the new schedule; none was sleeping even 8¼ hours on school nights.

"Even without the pressure of biological changes, if we combine an early school starting time—say 7:30 A.M., which, with a modest commute, makes 6:15 A.M. a viable rising time—with our knowledge that optimal sleep need is 9¼ hours, we are asking that 16-year olds go to bed at 9 P.M. Rare is a teenager that will keep such a schedule. School work, sports practices, clubs, volunteer work, and paid employment take precedence. When biological changes are factored in, the ability even to have merely 'adequate' sleep is lost," Carskadon explains.

♣ It's A Fact!!
Why Do Schools Have Such Early Start Times?

Given all the research that supports teenagers' sleep cycles, sleep needs and obstacles, students are still required to go to school at the crack of dawn, sometimes before 7 A.M. Most school districts have a delicately balanced bus transportation system designed to run as efficiently and inexpensively as possible. Using the same buses and drivers to bring all school age children to school saves money and helps distribute traffic during rush hours.

Another issue is after-school programming. Any delay in the start of school will result in a later release time. This reduces time (especially daylight hours) for practice and matches. Many high school students are involved in athletics, with matches and practice starting after school ends. If one school changes its start (and therefore end time) of school, students may have to miss class in order to make it to a match or game on time. In other cases, practice space is shared between schools and there will be more competition for field and gym space, which may result in the cancellation of some programs (such as JV and sports like swimming and golf, which often require the use of facilities during off-peak hours).

Some worry that a later start and release time will leave teachers with less time for their families. Teachers who have created a life around their current schedule may not want to come in and go home later.

Source: Excerpted from "Sleepiness in Teens: Not Just a Side Effect of Growing UP," © 2005 National Sleep Foundation (www.sleepfoundation.org). All rights reserved. Reprinted with permission.

School Start Time Initiatives and Outcomes

Minnesota (1996)

Early results from schools that have changed their start times are encouraging. For example, successful high school start time changes were made in Edina and Minneapolis, Minnesota after the Minnesota Medical Association issued a 1993 resolution, Sleep Deprivation in Adolescents, based on the research that puberty resets teens' internal biological clocks. The schedule was changed from:

- A 7:15 A.M.–1:45 P.M. day to an 8:40 A.M.–3:20 P.M. day in Minneapolis

- A 7:25 A.M.–2:10 P.M. day to an 8:30 A.M.–3:10 P.M. day in Edina

Results: The Center for Applied Research and Educational Improvement (CAREI) at the University of Minnesota conducted a study on the impact of changing school start times on academic performance, behavior and safety in urban and suburban schools (Wahlstrom, 2002). Results from three years of data from both Edina and Minneapolis showed:

- Improved attendance

- Increase in continuous enrollment

- Less tardiness

- Students making fewer trips to the school nurse

In suburban districts, students reported:

- Gaining an average of about one hour of sleep per night, since their bed times stayed the same even after the start time change.

- Eating breakfast more frequently.

- Being able to complete more of their homework during school hours, because they were more alert and efficient during the day.

Grades showed a slight improvement, although the change was not statistically significant. Researchers noted that it was difficult to assess changes in grades due to differences in school schedules, course names, grading policies, student transience, and the subjective nature of grading by teachers.

Suburban teachers and principals reported:

- Students seemed more alert in class.
- Improvements in student behavior, with a calmer atmosphere in the hallways and cafeteria.
- Fewer disciplinary referrals to the principal.

Suburban counselors reported:

- Fewer students seeking help for stress relief due to academic pressures.
- Fewer students coming to them with peer relationship problems and difficulties with parents.

Urban teachers, on the other hand, did not see any general improvement in student behavior.

In suburban schools, after-school athletic and other activity practices and rehearsals were shortened, with students arriving home later; however, actual participation in extracurricular activities and after-school jobs remained at the same level after the start time change. Urban schools, on the other hand, reported fewer students being involved in extracurricular activities, as well as conflicts with after-school jobs and compromised earnings. While some coaches whose sports involved long practices and traveling long distances for events disliked the change, most coaches and activity leaders supported the change because they felt students were less tired and more mentally alert at the end of the day.

Most suburban parents supported the change; urban parents had mixed reactions because of work schedules and transportation limitations. Both groups said their children were easier to live with, with fewer confrontations and more actual conversations and connecting time in the morning.

Massachusetts (2004)

Middle school students, many of whom are entering puberty and experiencing changes to their sleep patterns, have also benefited from later start times (Baroni et al., 2004). In a study comparing 7th and 8th graders at two different schools—one starting at 7:15 A.M., the other starting at 8:37 A.M.—the students who started school earlier reported inadequate sleep and struggling to stay awake in school more often than the students who started later. While there was no difference in weekend sleep patterns between the students at the two schools, the students who started school later reported sleeping an hour longer on school nights than those with early start times. This difference was due to later rise times; there was no difference in bed times. Academic benefits were also apparent, as students whose school started earlier were tardy four times more often, and 8th grade transcripts showed significantly worse grades. These results occurred in the fall following the start time change, and these findings were replicated in the spring. Although students at both schools were not getting enough sleep, the negative effects of sleep deprivation were far more pronounced in the earlier starting school.

Kentucky (1998): Preventing Drowsy Driving Crashes

Other school districts have focused on improved safety as a successful outcome of later start times. In fall 1998, a school district in Fayette County, Kentucky moved its start time from 7:30 A.M. to 8:30 A.M., and students averaged up to 50 minutes more sleep per night. Comparisons in the collision rates of Fayette County teens revealed that the crash rate for 16–18 year olds dropped following the change, even while crash rates for 17–18 year olds actually rose in the rest of the state.

This finding is especially important considering data from the National Highway Traffic Safety Administration, which estimates that up to 100,000 police-reported crashes annually are related to drowsiness, and that among drivers age 15–24, more than 1,500 fatalities each year are associated with such crashes. In a North Carolina state study, 55% of fall asleep crashes involved drivers 25 years old or younger.

Thus, unstable wakefulness and lapses in attention are not just detrimental to performance, like students missing an important piece of information from a teacher—they can also be dangerous, such as a sleepy driver missing a stop sign and causing a fatal accident.

Collaborating In The Best Interests Of Students

Many schools across the country are working to synchronize school clocks with students' body clocks, so that teens are in school during their most alert hours and can achieve their full academic potential. Working to bring school start times in line with teens' sleep needs presents a number of challenges and opportunities. Individual communities can vary greatly in their priorities and values; factors to consider include bell schedules of elementary and middle schools; transportation; athletic programs and extracurricular activities; use of schools for community activities; student employment; and safety issues for younger students who either may be waiting for a bus in the dark or need supervision of older siblings after school. There are also safety issues for older students, since violent activities, sex, recreational use of alcohol or drugs, and criminal and other risky behaviors frequently occur between 2 and 4 P.M., according to data from the Federal Bureau of Investigation. It is also important that any consideration of a school start time change takes into account the impact on families, including transportation, dependence on teens' income, chores and other family responsibilities, and teens' mood and behavior at home.

Changing a school's start time involves a wide array of people—parents, teachers, students, principals, school boards, superintendents, counselors, and healthcare professionals, among others. The impact is felt at a community level, but it is also felt individually, and the individuals who are affected need to have their views heard and acknowledged so that discussions can move forward in search of common ground.

Remember!!

Obviously, moving bell times is one major step in a larger picture of ensuring that adolescents get the sleep they need. It will not put more hours in the day, so it is important for teens to know about their sleep needs and have the skills to make a conscious effort to get a good night's sleep. Many teens assume they are expected to function with a lack of sleep, but sleep is not optional; it is biologically necessary. If sleep is incorporated into educational efforts, teens will be armed with information that will enable them to use a later school start time to their advantage.

Source: "Backgrounder: Research, Advocacy, Later Start Times," © 2007 National Sleep Foundation.

Chapter 40

Sleep May Be Critical For Biochemical Brain Processes

Sleep can be wonderfully restorative. After a long day of work you drag your-self to bed—and then you wake up seven or eight hours later, alert and recharged.

Now, researchers are finding that one reason we sleep may be that our brains, as well as our bodies, need time to rest and repair themselves. Recent studies have suggested that the brain, so active during the day, may use the downtime of sleep to repair damage caused by our busy metabolism, replen-ish dwindling energy stores, and even grow new neurons.

These studies, along with competing and complementary research on sleep and memory and the evolutionary forces driving sleep, are giving us a fuller picture of the biological imperatives behind this most basic need.

Messy Metabolism

One way that sleep may aid the brain is by reducing damage caused by oxidative stress. For years, researchers have known that molecules called free radicals can damage human cells, including brain cells. These molecules form naturally whenever the body metabolizes oxygen, so the damage they cause is called oxidative stress. Because free radicals are missing one electron, they're very unstable and bind to other molecules in nerve cells and elsewhere—and when they do they damage those cells.

The body combats free radicals with neutralizing enzymes, including one called superoxide dismutase (SOD) that can break down the damaging molecules into their component, and harmless, parts. But research has found that when a rat is sleep-deprived the level of SOD in its brain drops, suggesting that sleep may be crucial for minimizing the brain cell damage caused by oxidative stress, says study author Jerome Siegel, PhD, a psychologist at the University of California, Los Angeles.

In the 2002 study, published in the journal *Neuroreport* (Vol. 13, No. 11, pages 1,387–1,390), Siegel and his colleagues kept rats awake for five to 11 days. At the end of the sleep deprivation period, they found that the level of SOD activity had decreased in the rats' hippocampus and brainstem.

In another 2002 study, this one in the journal *Brain Research* (Vol. 945, No. 1, pages 1–8), Siegel's team found some evidence of the effect that this reduced SOD activity might have caused damage to cell membranes in the hypothalamus of rats kept awake for 45 hours in a row.

Free radicals can also damage other cells in the body. But other types of tissue—like muscles—can rest any time we sit still, Siegel explains. The brain, on the other hand, is hard at work whenever we're awake.

"Putting these together, the message is that sleep deprivation causes oxidative stress in the brain, and in the regions where the stress is more severe, it causes damage," he says. On the other hand, he points out, the cells in his study were damaged but not dead—so some of the damage might be reversible with sleep. The results also fit with what we know about animal sleep, Siegel adds. In general, smaller animals require more sleep than larger ones. Smaller animals also generally have a higher metabolic rate—which would produce more free radicals, and thus necessitate more sleep to neutralize them.

The Brain's Battery

All that messy metabolism requires energy to keep running. And over the past decade or so, several researchers have suggested that another purpose of sleep might be to replenish the energy stores that we use up while awake.

Harvard Medical School neuroscientist Robert McCarley, MD, studies the link between sleep and a molecule called adenosine triphosphate (ATP), which provides energy to cells. ATP stores energy in the chemical bonds that hold it together, and when it breaks down into its component parts it releases that energy to the cell. One of those component parts is the neurotransmitter adenosine, which McCarley and others now think the brain may use as a signal to monitor its need for sleep.

In a 1997 study published in *Science* (Vol. 276, No. 5316, pages 1,265–1,268), McCarley and his colleagues measured the level of adenosine in the brains of cats kept awake for six hours—much longer than a cat would naturally stay awake. The researchers found that the level of adenosine in the cat's basal forebrain—an important area for regulating sleep and wake—increased with each hour of sleep deprivation.

In a 2000 follow-up study, published in *Neuroscience* (Vol. 99, No. 3, pages 507–517), the researchers found that this was not true in other areas of the brain—such as the cerebral cortex—that were less important for regulating sleep.

The idea, then, is that this is a self-regulating cycle. As the level of ATP in brain cells drops, the level of adenosine rises. That rising level of adenosine sends a signal to the areas of the brain that regulate sleep that it's time to sleep.

"Adenosine is the messenger telling the cell to shut off—that you need some rest," McCarley says.

Other researchers have suggested other possible contenders for the substance linking energy to sleep. Neuroscientists Joel Benington, PhD, of St. Bonaventure University, and Craig Heller, PhD, of Stanford University, were among the first to suggest that energy restoration in the brain might be a function of sleep. They focused on glycogen, a form of glucose that provides energy to localized brain cells when they need a short-term boost.

Studies, though, have provided mixed results. While researchers have found that levels of glycogen dip in the brain after sleep deprivation in some strains of mice, other strains haven't shown that expected pattern.

"It's a mixed bag of results, with nothing conclusive yet," says Benington.

Neurogenesis

Other research suggests that sleep may contribute to neurogenesis, or the formation of new nerve cells in the brain.

For decades, scientists believed that animals and humans were born with all the brain cells they would ever have. Over the past 30 years, though, neuroscientists have chipped away at that theory, finding evidence of new brain cell growth first in adult rats, then in primates, and finally, in the late 1990s, in humans—particularly in an area of the hippocampus called the dentate gyrus.

But recent evidence shows that sleep deprivation can impede these new neurons' growth. In a 2003 study in the *Journal of Physiology* (Vol. 549, No. 2, pages 563–571), neuroscientist Dennis McGinty, PhD, and his colleagues at the University of California, Los Angeles, found that depriving rats of sleep for four days reduced the number of new cells in the dentate gyrus by more than 50 percent.

In a follow-up study published in October in the *European Journal of Neuroscience* (Vol. 22, No. 8, pages 2,111–2,116), they found that many cells that formed during sleep-deprivation didn't mature normally.

"The nice thing about this model is that it's very concrete," McGinty says. "People have wanted for years to understand how sleep could play a role in brain development and growth, and this gives you a direct way to look at structural change."

Overall, McGinty points out, it's important to remember that most of the hypothesized functions of sleep—reducing oxidative stress, restoring energy levels, promoting neurogenesis, and others—are not mutually exclusive. In fact, many complement each other.

"Even something as simple as breathing has multiple functions," he says. "So it's quite likely that something as complex as sleep is in the same boat."

Chapter 41

Research Confirms The Virtues of "Sleeping On It"

Recent studies show that both slow-wave and rapid eye movement (REM) sleep are important for consolidating learning and memory—and perhaps even for solving intractable problems.

Researchers have increasingly recognized, in recent years, that sleep serves many functions, including providing an opportunity for the body to rest, facilitating metabolic and endocrine function, and enabling "offline" memory processing. Still, the mechanisms underlying these functions have remained remarkably mysterious.

"Of all the biological drives—such as thirst, hunger, and sexual desire—sleep is the only one whose function wasn't obvious 2,000 years ago," observes Robert Stickgold, PhD, a cognitive neuroscientist at the Harvard Medical School and the Massachusetts Mental Health Center.

In the case of sleep's effect on learning and memory, for example, studies have produced conflicting results over the years, with some linking REM sleep, in particular, to improved memory, and others failing to find such effects.

But recent investigations have yielded new insight into sleep's role in memory and learning. The research confirms what some sleep experts have long theorized: that sleep is critical for firming up the learning that took place during the day—a process known as memory consolidation.

In two recent studies, Stickgold and his colleagues tested people's learning on a standard test of perceptual memory known as a visual discrimination task. They first trained study participants to perform the discrimination task as quickly as possible, then measured how well participants had learned the procedure by testing their improvement on the task hours later.

> ♣ **It's A Fact!!**
>
> Recent findings call for "a changing view of memory, not just as storage but as a way of learning from experience, re-organizing thinking and building models of the world. If we can think of sleep as a creative learning process that allows us to extrapolate and look for novel juxtapositions of events, clearly that would be valu-able in terms of our use of memory." —Matthew A. Wilson, Massachusetts Institute of Technology

In an article published in the *Journal of Cognitive Neuroscience* (Vol. 12, No. 2) in March 2000, the researchers reported that participants showed no improvement when they were tested on the same day on which they had been trained. But when people had slept for at least six hours after training and before testing, they showed consistent improvement on the discrimination task.

In addition, the study showed that the amount of improvement that participants demonstrated was directly proportional to the amount of slow-wave sleep that they obtained early in the night and the amount of REM sleep that they obtained late in the night. In fact, Stickgold's group found that the amount of sleep that participants got during these two phases accounted for a striking 80 percent of the difference among participants in improvement on the visual discrimination task.

"That was startling to us," says Stickgold. "I've never seen such a strong correlation between the quality of people's sleep and any behavioral measures, let alone measures of memory and learning."

A further investigation, published in the journal *Nature Neuroscience* (Vol. 3, No. 12) in December 2000, found that a single night of sleep deprivation permanently short-circuited the memory-consolidation process: Participants who had been kept awake for 30 hours after an initial training session showed no evidence of improved performance on the visual discrimination test, even after two nights of restorative sleep.

In related research published in the journal *Science* (Vol. 290) in October 2000, Stickgold and colleagues had participants play the computer game "Tetris" for seven hours over the course of three days. They found that when research participants were awakened just after they fell asleep, 75 percent reported experiencing visual images of the game, suggesting that they were continuing to work on the problem during sleep.

"This is what 'sleeping on a problem' is all about," says Stickgold. He speculates that slow-wave and REM sleep activate a sort of "primal calculation mechanism" that helps the brain extract meaning from jumbled information.

Further support for that view comes from recent research on memory consolidation in rats by Massachusetts Institute of Technology neuroscientist Matthew A. Wilson, PhD, and colleagues. Two studies, published in the journal *Neuron* in November 1998 and January 2001 (Vol. 21, No. 5 and Vol. 29, No. 1, respectively), revealed the same patterns of brain activation when rats were learning to navigate in a maze and during subsequent slow-wave and REM sleep.

Such evidence of recently learned material being "replayed" during sleep is consistent with recent research in humans, led by Pierre Maquet, MD, a neuroscientist at the University of Liège, Belgium, and published in the journal *Nature Neuroscience* (Vol. 3, No. 8) in August 2000. Using positron emission tomography to trace brain activity, Maquet's group found that the brain areas that were activated when participants were learning a serial reaction time task were also activated during subsequent REM sleep.

Like Wilson's research, those findings appear to confirm that "what one learned earlier is being replayed and rehearsed, and the [memory] circuits are becoming stronger," says Carlyle Smith, PhD, a biopsychologist at Trent University in Peterborough, Ontario, and one of Maquet's co-authors.

Together, agrees Wilson, the recent findings call for "a changing view of memory, not just as storage but as a way of learning from experience, reorganizing thinking and building models of the world.

"If we can think of sleep as a creative learning process that allows us to extrapolate and look for novel juxtapositions of events, clearly that would be valuable in terms of our use of memory."

Chapter 42

A Biomarker In Saliva May Help Measure Sleep Deprivation

If a jolty ride on public transportation has ever left you wondering whether the driver was dozing off at the wheel, consider the results of a new study that suggests sleepiness might one day be measured by taking a saliva sample.

The study, published in the Proceedings of the National Academy of Sciences[1], identifies a chemical in saliva whose levels go up when people are sleep-deprived and down when they are rested. The chemical could be used as a "biomarker" to gauge sleepiness in a variety of occupational settings where tired workers are likely to put themselves and others at risk, said the study's senior author, Paul J. Shaw, Ph.D., a professor of anatomy and neuro-biology at Washington University School of Medicine in St. Louis.

Dr. Shaw's work and other studies on the basic mechanisms of sleep fill an important public health need, said Merrill Mitler, Ph.D., a program di-rector in the Division of Extramural Research at the National Institute of Neurological Disorders and Stroke (NINDS).

"Excessive sleepiness troubles millions of Americans. It can be the result of sleep apnea or another disorder, a side effect of medication, or simply the product of a demanding work schedule," Dr. Mitler said. "Whatever the

About This Chapter: "Sure You're Awake? Spit into this Cup," National Institute of Neurological Disorders and Stroke, March 9, 2007.

cause, insufficient sleep can create significant health risks, both for the affected person and others."

Among the many situations where a lack of sleep could be dangerous, driving stands out as the most statistically relevant. Sleep deprivation among medical personnel, especially young residents, has become a major concern at hospitals. Indeed, sleep-related accidents have generated a spate of malpractice lawsuits, leading some hospitals to impose tighter limits over the hours their residents work.

An obvious way to find out if people are sleep-deprived is to ask them, or to look for visible signs of sleepiness (bloodshot eyes, slurred speech, poor attention). But these approaches often miss the truth, said Dr. Shaw.

♣ **It's A Fact!!**
The National Highway Traffic Safety Administration estimates that sleepiness may be a factor in 20 percent of motor vehicle crashes, some of which probably can be traced to the long hours that truckers are expected to spend behind the wheel.

"People tend not to admit they're tired," he said. "And the overt signs that someone is sleepy tend to happen long after he's already in trouble. We want to identify people who are tired before something bad happens."

Dr. Shaw, who is supported by NINDS, began his search for a biomarker of sleepiness in fruit flies. Although they can do it clinging to a wall, flies sleep in a manner reminiscent of other animals, he said. They become quiet and still for about 90 minutes at a time, sleeping about 12 hours total each day. Their well-characterized genetics, and the ability to study mutant flies with altered sleep behavior, facilitated Dr. Shaw's search.

Dr. Shaw first used a DNA microarray to scan for genes whose activity was altered in sleep-deprived flies. Activity of the gene encoding amylase consistently spiked in flies that were kept awake.

In another set of experiments, Dr. Shaw measured the activity of the amylase gene relative to the flies' sleep patterns by probing for amylase RNA. He showed that amylase RNA levels increase specifically prior to a condition known as "sleep rebound." The experiments were important for establishing amylase as a biomarker for sleepiness, he said, because many genes might be expected to turn on in an awake fly (or person), even one that isn't feeling sleepy.

Dr. Shaw collaborated with Stephen Duntley, M.D., a professor of neurology at Washington University's Sleep Medicine Center, to determine if amylase levels are a surrogate for sleepiness in people. Nine volunteers were monitored at the sleep center during a weekend of normal sleep, and during a weekend when they went without sleep for 28 hours. Amylase RNA was probed in the participants' saliva. Drs. Shaw and Duntley found that in people, as in flies, the RNA levels climbed during sleep deprivation.

In addition to identifying people who are at risk for sleep-related accidents, Dr. Shaw speculated that amylase levels in saliva could be used to measure sleepiness in research on the mechanisms of sleep. The need for sleep varies widely among people and among animal species, he said, and a biomarker for sleepiness could help researchers sort out the genetic basis for those differences. Electroencephalography (EEG) can be used to record brain waves that herald the onset of sleep, but the technique is time-consuming and not always practical.

"It's hard to put electrodes on a killer whale," Dr. Shaw said, noting that whales can go for extended periods without sleeping.

"Our immediate goal is to shift the focus away from amylase toward identifying other biomarkers," he said. A panel of biomarkers could be cross-checked against each other, he explained, giving researchers the most accurate assessments of when people, flies, and other creatures are in need of a good night's sleep.

✎ What's It Mean?

Amylase: A protein in animal saliva that helps digest starch.

Amylase RNA: The chemical intermediate necessary to convert the amylase gene into protein.

DNA Microarray: A chip coated with thousands of genetic probes.

Sleep Rebound: A period of deep slumbering that satisfies the need for sleep.

Reference

1. Seugnet L, Boero J, Gottschalk L, Duntley SP, and Shaw PJ. "Identification of a Biomarker for Sleep Drive in Flies and Humans." *Proceedings of the National Academy of Sciences*. December 26, 2006, Vol. 103(52), pp. 19913–19918.

Chapter 43

Histamine Is Key To Wakefulness

Scientists studying an animal model of narcolepsy have found that hista-
mine-activated brain cells are key to wakefulness. The study was funded in
part by the National Institute of Neurological Disorders and Stroke (NINDS)
and appeared in the journal *Neuron*.[1]

Narcolepsy is a disorder of sleep regulation that affects control of wakefulness and sleep and renders the patient subject to disabling sleepiness during the day. Some patients also have episodes of cataplexy, in which they
suddenly lose muscle tone and go limp for up to 30 seconds but remains fully
conscious. Cataplexy resembles wakefulness in that consciousness is preserved
and also resembles Rapid Eye Movement (REM) sleep—a deep sleep in
which most of our dreams occur—in that the individual loses muscle tone.

Researchers previously thought that brain cells that use serotonin, norepinephrine, and histamine to transmit nerve impulses acted identically in
regulating sleep and arousal, with chemical levels being high during wakefulness and reduced during sleep.

Studying dogs that are specially bred to carry a genetic form of narcolepsy,
lead investigator Jerome Siegel, Ph.D., of the University of California-Los

About This Chapter: "Study in Dogs Shows that Histamine is Key to Wakefulness,"
National Institute of Neurological Disorders and Stroke, September 2004.

Angeles, and colleagues examined histamine brain cell activity when the dogs were in cataplexy and during REM sleep. The team found that histamine neuron activity continued during cataplexy but ceased during sleep, showing that the chemical was key to waking. The scientists also found that serotonin and norepinephrine neuron activity were high during wakefulness but shut off during sleep and cataplexy, causing the loss of muscle tone seen in both conditions.

The findings also show why antihistamines, commonly used to treat colds and allergies, cause drowsiness and impair alertness.

"Our findings greatly improve our understanding of the brain activity responsible for maintaining consciousness and muscle tone while awake," said Dr. Siegel. "These findings should aid in the development of drugs to induce sleep and increase alertness."

"These findings are interesting both scientifically and pharmacologically," said Merrill Mitler, Ph.D., NINDS' program director for sleep research. "Many over the counter sleep remedies currently contain antihistamines and can be quite sedating, but don't necessarily promote natural sleep. A better understanding of the chemical interactions involved with wakefulness and sleep may lead to new treatments that counter daytime sleepiness and offer satisfying sleep for persons with sleep problems such as insomnia."

✎ What's It Mean?

Histamine: A neurotransmitter and hormone that occurs naturally in the body. Histamine-containing neurons are found in the hypothalamus and project into the areas of the brain that are involved with sleep, memory, emotion, and temperature.

Reference

1. John J, We M-F, Boehmer L, Siegel JM. "Cataplexy-Active Neurons in the Hypothalamus: Implications for the Role of Histamine in Sleep and Waking Behavior." Neuron, Vol. 42, May 27, 2004, pp. 619–634.

Chapter 44

Sleep Research At The National Institutes Of Health

Introduction

The Trans-NIH Sleep Research Coordinating Committee (SRCC) was established in 1986 by the Director, National Institutes of Health (NIH) for the purpose of facilitating interchange of information on sleep and sleep-related research. In conjunction with the creation of National Center on Sleep Disorders Research (NCSDR) in 1993, the Director of NIH transferred responsibility for the Trans-NIH SRCC to the NCSDR, and the NCSDR Director serves as Chair of the Trans-NIH SRCC.

The NCSDR is a component of the National Heart, Lung, and Blood Institute (NHLBI) and is charged with the conduct and support of research, training, health information dissemination, and other activities with respect to sleep disorders, including biological and circadian rhythm research, basic

About This Chapter: This chapter includes excerpts from "Annual Report of the Trans-NIH Sleep Research Coordinating Committee, Fiscal Year 2005," National Heart, Lung, and Blood Institute (NHLBI). The full text of this report is available online at http://www.nhlbi.nih.gov/health/prof/sleep/sleep-05.htm. Supplemental information in call-out boxes identified as "NHLBI, 2004" was excerpted from "Annual Report of the Trans-NIH Sleep Research Coordinating Committee, Fiscal Year 2004," NHLBI. The full text of this reports is available online at http://www.nhlbi.nih.gov/health/prof/sleep/sleep-04.htm.

understanding of sleep, chronobiological and other sleep related research. The NCSDR also coordinates the activities of the Center with similar activities of other federal agencies, including the other agencies of the NIH, and similar activities of other public and nonprofit entities.

National Center On Sleep Disorders Research

NCSDR maintains a website (http://www.nhlbi.nih.gov/sleep) with information on sleep disorders for patients and health care providers. A special area of emphasis is educating youth. The NCSDR Sleep Well, Do Well, Star Sleeper Campaign (http://www.nhlbi.nih.gov/health/public/sleep/starslp) was launched in 2001 and continues to educate America's children—and their parents, educators, and healthcare providers—about the importance of adequate night time sleep.

> **✤ It's A Fact!!**
>
> The field of sleep medicine is multidisciplinary, cutting across multiple Institutes and Centers of the National Institutes of Health (NIH). Sleep research is not limited to very young and old patients—sleep disorders reach across all ages and ethnicities.
>
> Source: NHLBI, 2004.

NCSDR convened two meetings of the Sleep Disorders Research Advisory Board including representatives from other federal agencies in Fiscal Year 2005 to discuss the status of sleep disorders research. These meetings are videocast live and accessible in an online archive at http://www.videocast.nih.gov/PastEvents.asp?c=26

National Heart, Lung, And Blood Institute

The NHLBI sleep research program covers a spectrum of sleep research related to heart, lung, and blood diseases. The research programs are aimed at understanding the molecular, genetic, and physiological underpinnings of sleep and sleep disorders through basic, clinical, and epidemiological research. A major focus is sleep disordered breathing (SDB) as a potential risk factor for cardiopulmonary disease, stroke, and weight gain. NHLBI is a major supporter of investigator-initiated sleep research at NIH.

Mounting evidence indicates that SDB is a chronic disease condition associated with serious cardiovascular outcomes. Evidence suggests that SDB is relatively common affecting at least 3% of children, 2% of middle-aged women, 4% of middle-aged men, and 10–20% of the elderly. The incidence of new sleep disordered breathing cases has been estimated to be 3–6%. However, less than 10% of adult SDB cases are diagnosed. If left untreated, SDB predisposes to an increased risk of new hypertension and heart. Since the treatment of SDB may ameliorate the severity of cardiovascular disease risk factors, studies of the relationship between SDB and cardiovascular outcomes are clinically important.

Stroke: New findings from two independent studies associate SDB with a 2–4 fold increased frequency of stroke in middle age adults. The association was independent of common risk factors including age, sex, race, smoking status, body-mass index (BMI), and the presence or absence of diabetes mellitus, hyperlipidemia, atrial fibrillation, and hypertension. This is the first longitudinal study indicating that the relationship of sleep apnea severity to stroke and all-cause mortality is independent of common cardiovascular and cerebrovascular risk factors.

♣ It's A Fact!!

Evidence links both too little and too much sleep to an increased risk of mortality [death] and morbidity [disease]. A study of over 3,000 women demonstrates that the risk of death is three times greater among those who sleep more or less than the average of 6–8 hours per night. Daytime sleepiness also appears linked to mortality. The results suggest that each hour of napping is associated with a 6% increased risk of mortality. Women reporting daily naps also walk slower and exhibit weaker hand grip strength. Difficulty sleeping or functioning due to poor sleep (34% of women at baseline) was associated with a two times greater risk of depressive symptoms at follow up.

Source: NHLBI, 2004.

Left Ventricular Function In Children: A recent study evaluated heart function in children (ages 5–18) referred to a pediatric sleep clinic. Left ventricular (LV) diastolic function was decreased in apneic children compared to children with very mild sleep disordered breathing (snoring). The decrease in LV function was proportional to apnea severity and independent of age, gender, race, and blood pressure. Follow-up of 10 children in which the apnea was treated and managed for one year (tonsillectomy, uvulopalatopharyngoplasty, or CPAP dictated by standard of care) revealed an 18% improvement in LV function.

Short Sleep Duration, Metabolism Impairment, And Elevated Risk of Obesity: New findings from the Sleep Heart Health Study indicate that sleep duration of six hours or less is associated with an increased frequency of diabetes and impaired glucose tolerance (IGT). At five hours of sleep or less, the odds ratio for diabetes presence increased to 2.5, and with six hours of sleep the odds ratio for diabetes presence increased to 1.6 compared to those with 7–8 hours of sleep. The association between sleep duration and IGT and diabetes persists after excluding insomnia and adjusting for girth, demographic factors, caffeine, and cardiovascular disease risk factors. Sleep duration longer than 9 hours per night was also associated with a greater risk of poor glycemic control.

New findings also link insufficient sleep to abnormalities in the regulation of hunger, satiety, and metabolism. Mice with a mutation in the Clock gene sleep less, expend less energy, consume more calories, and gain as much weight on a regular diet as normal mice fed a high-fat diet. Overall daily activity levels in mutant and normal mice are similar. Short sleeping mutant mice fed a high-fat diet gained about 50% more weight than normal mice on this diet. The adult short sleeping mutant mice had high levels of blood cholesterol, triglycerides, and glucose, and insulin resistance indicative of metabolic disease. High leptin blood levels and reduced levels of ghrelin and orexin in brain indicate that abnormalities in signaling satiety and hunger to brain are associated with weight gain in the short sleeping mutant mice.

Future Directions: Voluntary sleep curtailment (habitual short sleep duration) is a pervasive lifestyle and untreated sleep disorders are also common. Average sleep duration in adults has declined from 8.5 to less than 7 hours/

> ## ♣ It's A Fact!!
>
> Sleep medicine and sleep research have been growing exponentially during the last 20 years. By 2002, over 2,000 specialized sleep centers existed in the United States. The growth of the field has been fueled by the needs of a large patient population. Although clinical practice related to sleep problems and sleep disorders has been expanding rapidly in the last few years, scientific research is not keeping pace. Insomnia and restless legs syndrome are two examples of very common disorders about which very little is known neurobiologically. Treatments for sleep apnea (for example, continuous positive airway pressure) have made a huge difference in the lives of many patients, yet they are still fairly intrusive and not universally accepted by patients.
>
> Source: NHLBI, 2004.

night over the last 40 years. Typical sleep durations of six hours are now common and the proportion of young adults sleeping less than seven hours has increased from 16 to 37%. Declines in sleep duration have occurred concurrent with an upward trend in obesity prevalence, but only recently have sufficient data emerged to suggest that these two epidemics may have mechanistic interrelationships. Studies are needed to elucidate cause-and-effect relationships and mechanisms to explain associations between short sleep duration and increased risk of obesity or overweight due to altered metabolism, appetite, or inflammation.

National Institute On Aging

Sleep is essential to well-being and occupies about a third of our lives. Without enough sleep, fatigue, clouded thinking, possible metabolic dysregulation leading to diabetes and obesity, and diminished quality of life can occur. For older people, these symptoms can be more than a matter of discomfort; they can lead to more serious complications. Falls resulting from fatigue and confusion, for example, can result in debilitating, costly injuries in this vulnerable population. The importance of recognizing and treating age-associated health problems, such as sleep disorders, takes on new dimension as the nation's elderly population grows to record numbers.

Many people believe that poor sleep is a normal part of aging, but it is not. In fact, many healthy older adults report few or no sleep problems. Sleep patterns change as we age, but disturbed sleep and waking up tired everyday are not part of normal aging. However, many older adults have sleep problems, which are often linked to underlying medical conditions. Abnormal sleep can cause disease; but diseases can cause abnormal sleep. Changes in daily sleep patterns are some of the most prominent behavioral and symptomatic changes that occur with aging. Understanding the age-related changes in the nervous system that underlie changes in sleep can lead to better means of primary and secondary prevention of these disorders and, thus, reduce the economic and social impacts of sleep disturbances in the older population.

Health Disparities Related Research: Sleep disordered breathing (SDB) is a highly prevalent sleep disorder in older persons. Differences in SDB between people with hypertension (high blood pressure) with or without a family history of hypertension were studied in African Americans. Increasing weight was accompanied by increasing severity of SDB. Hypertensives with a family history are likely to show a profile of greater blood pressure, higher body mass index (BMI), and more severe SDB, which are more common among African Americans.

Individuals of lower individual and household education were significantly more likely to experience insomnia even after controlling for ethnicity, gender, and age. Additionally, individuals with fewer years of education, particularly those who had dropped out of high school, experienced greater subjective impairment because of their insomnia.

Neuroimaging: The use of neuroimaging technologies to study sleep is relatively new. In general, studies have found that there is a global decrease in brain activity during non-rapid eye movement (NREM) sleep, suggesting a down-regulation of the central nervous system (CNS) with deepening sleep. During REM sleep, however, there appears to be an increase in metabolic activity, which could be linked to the dream activity that is concentrated during REM sleep. Using positron emission tomography (PET) technology, it has recently been reported that patients with insomnia show greater global glucose cerebral metabolism during sleep and while awake, than do normal sleepers, and that there is a smaller decline in the metabolism of the wake-promoting regions of the brain during the transition from wake to sleep, suggesting that the disturbed sleep of insomnia is associated with a failure of arousal mechanisms to decrease sufficiently while transitioning to sleep. Furthermore, there was reduced daytime metabolic activity in the prefrontal cortex resulting from the insomnia.

Hypertension: Some sleep disorders have been linked to hypertension, but few studies have examined the relationship between daytime sleepiness and blood pressure. A recent study determined that scores on a short questionnaire assessing daytime sleepiness (Epworth Sleepiness Scale [ESS]) were associated with blood pressure and could be used to predict hypertension after five years in healthy older adults, men and women 55 to 80 years of age, who had not previously been diagnosed with hypertension. Compared to individuals with low ESS sores, those scoring high had increased casual and sleep blood pressure as well as higher systolic blood pressure levels and diastolic blood pressure variability during waking hours, and reported higher levels of anger, depression, anxiety, and intensity of psychological symptoms as well as lower defensiveness. Individuals with high ESS scores were more likely to be diagnosed with hypertension five years later. Groups with high and low ESS scores did not differ significantly on any other variables. The ESS, a simple measure of daytime sleepiness, identified individuals at risk for hypertension. Future studies should investigate the possibility that diagnosis and treatment of daytime sleepiness could aid in blood pressure reduction and ultimately in decreased morbidity and mortality from cardiovascular disorders. Reduction of sleep times may lead to metabolic dysfunctions leading to obesity, hypertension, insulin resistance, and a diabetic phenotype.

Metabolism: Leptin and ghrelin are two hormones that provide the brain information about energy balance. Leptin, produced by adipocytes (fat cells), rapidly increases when there is an excess of caloric intake and decreases appetite. In contrast, ghrelin, produced primarily in the stomach, stimulates appetite. In experimental studies carbohydrate metabolism, endocrine function, and gastrointestinal balance in young, healthy adults were studied after restricting sleep to four hours per night for six nights as compared to a fully rested condition. Leptin levels were decreased, ghrelin levels were increased, and there was an increase in hunger and appetite under the short sleep condition with levels of activity and caloric intake the same for both conditions.

This was associated with decreased glucose tolerance and insulin sensitivity and elevated evening cortisol levels.

Similar findings were found in a population-based longitudinal study of over a 1,000 participants now between 45 and 75 years of age. In those who slept less than 8 hours per night (about 75% of the sample), body mass index increased as sleep time decreased. Short sleep also was associated with reduced leptin and elevated ghrelin levels in the blood.

Circadian Rhythms: Other factors associated with aging, such as disease, changes in environment, or concurrent age-related processes may contribute to problems of sleep in older persons. Studies on young adults have shown that entrainment of the circadian timing system can be achieved with much lower light intensities than was previously estimated; light of indoor intensity can have a significant phase-shifting effect on the circadian pace-maker, and can suppress plasma melatonin secretion . Therefore, awakening early in the morning, such as when associated with nocturia (nighttime voiding), and turning on a lamp, may lead to an earlier entrainment of the circadian clock and contribute to the early morning awakenings of older individuals.

> **✤ It's A Fact!!**
> There has been an increasing trend towards shorter sleep times over the last century, and this has been mirrored by an increasing trend of obesity in the U.S. Studies now are showing that chronic sleep restriction is associated with hormonal and metabolic changes leading to the possible development of chronic conditions, such as obesity, diabetes, and hypertension, leading to increased cardiovascular disease morbidity and mortality. It now is clear that maintenance of proper sleep habits is necessary for the maintenance of health.
>
> Source: NHLBI, 2005.

Older adults with dementia often have disruptions in circadian rhythms, including disruptions of the rest-activity rhythm. Sleep disturbance is a symptom shared by all neurodegenerative, dementing illnesses, such as Alzheimer disease (AD) and dementia with Lewy bodies (DLB), and its presence frequently precipitates decisions to seek institutional care for patients. However, the consequences of disturbed rhythms are unknown. Patients with dementia appear to develop an abnormal timing of their rhythms, which is predictive of shorter survival.

Basic Mechanisms: An interesting recently discovered molecule is hypocretin (Hcrt), a hypothalamus-specific peptide. Two forms have been identified, Hcrt1 and Hcrt2, with the latter proposed as a peptide neurotransmitter. The brain cells that secrete the hypocretins make connections with many of the brain regions involved in regulating the sleep-wake cycle. The hypocretins may act as chemical signals involved in the mechanisms of homeostasis and alertness.

Future Directions: New studies are pursuing leads into the genetics of sleep. Similar to other recent findings that neuronal loss is not an inevitable consequence of aging, these data indicate that there is little evidence of an age-related loss of neurons that have been identified as playing a key role in the maintenance of sleep homeostasis. Thus, the age-related alterations in the control of sleep appear to not be due to loss of critical neurons but to subtle changes within the cells and in their interactions with other brain cells involved in the control of sleep and alertness. The clarification of these factors, such as the role played by adenosine in the induction of sleep, can lead to the development of more effective and targeted medications to alleviate some of the problems of sleep that afflict over half of our older population.

Research also needs to be directed at the development of new and more effective treatments that are targeted at correcting the underlying mechanisms of sleep disorders rather than treating symptoms. However, until that time, clinical trials on the safety and efficacy of sleep medications are still needed.

A large proportion of older nursing home residents have problems in nighttime sleep and daytime wake. They often are treated for their sleep problems with medications that may put them at risk for falls and confusion. Behavioral and environmental approaches may be more effective at dealing with these sleep problems, along with the identification of undiagnosed sleep apnea that could underlie some of these problems.

Research needs to further study the changes in sleep quality that occur through the adult age span and how these changes also mark specific alterations in hormonal systems that are essential for metabolic regulation. Sleep loss may increase the stress load, possibly facilitating the development of chronic conditions, such as obesity, diabetes, and hypertension, which have an increased prevalence in low socio-economic groups.

Another exciting area of newly developing research is the understanding of the relationships between sleep and cognitive functioning. This may be especially important in the older individual, given the increased risks for disturbed sleep and disturbed cognition.

♣ It's A Fact!!
Sleep Problems In Early Childhood
As A Risk Marker For Early Onset of Alcohol Abuse

It is well documented that sleep problems, primarily insomnia, are associated with the onset of alcohol problems among some adults and predict relapse in adult alcoholics in remission. In contrast, there are only a few studies in adolescents that have found a positive correlation between sleep disturbances and the presence of alcohol and other drug problems. Furthermore, because these studies in adolescents were cross-sectional and not prospective, it could not be determined whether sleep problems are the cause or consequence of drinking. However, a recent study has used a longitudinal prospective design to examine the relationship between sleep problems in early childhood and the onset of alcohol and other drug use in early adolescence. In this study, mothers' ratings of their children's sleep problems at ages 3 to 5 years significantly predicted an early onset of any use of alcohol, marijuana, and illicit drugs, as well as an early onset of cigarette use by age 12 to 14. Although sleep problems in early childhood also predicted attention problems and anxiety/depression in later childhood, these disorders did not mediate the relationship between sleep problems and the onset of alcohol and other drug use. This is the first study to demonstrate that early childhood sleep problems may be a marker for increased risk of later alcohol and drug use disorders.

Source: NHLBI, 2004.

National Institute On Alcohol Abuse And Alcoholism

Alcohol consumption and abuse leads to problems falling asleep, decrease in total sleep time, and disruptions in other biological rhythms. Recent research has investigated the effects of prenatal and adult alcohol exposure on circadian rhythmic output and the mechanisms underlying these changes.

Effects Of Alcohol On Circadian Activity Rhythms: Two studies examined the effects of chronic alcohol consumption and alcohol withdrawal on circadian rhythms of free-running activity and light responsiveness of the circadian pacemaker in adult rats. Results indicate that both chronic alcohol intake and alcohol withdrawal may produce changes in a fundamental parameter of the circadian pacemaker and its free-running period. In addition, chronic alcohol consumption may also affect the response of the circadian pacemaker to light signals.

Alcohol Effects On Central Clocks Controlling Neuroendocrine Function: Recent studies have shown that alcohol consumption affects the circadian functions of endorphin-containing neurons that are involved in control of reward and reinforcement in alcohol drinking. Chronic alcohol exposure causes major alterations in the central and internal clocks governing neuroendocrine functions and may have significant disease-related consequences.

Sleep Disturbance, Alcoholism Risk, And Remission: Two recent studies investigated the association of sleep disturbance with the following: 1) risk for alcohol-related problems, and 2) chronic dependence or remission of alcohol dependence. In the first study, it was found that individuals who report sleep disturbances because of worry are at increased risk of developing alcohol-related problems after an extended interval. Risk is highest among those with a history of anxiety disorders or mood symptoms. The exact pathway between sleep disturbances and alcohol-related problems is unknown. However, these findings emphasize the need to assess and treat sleep disturbances in those with psychiatric disorders, because of the potential to increase alcohol intake for self-medication of sleep problems.

In the second study, it was found that alcohol dependent individuals who reside in the community are twice as likely to self-report insomnia compared to those without a history of dependence. These findings underscore the importance for evaluation and treatment of sleep disturbances in individuals with persistent alcohol dependence, since sleep difficulties may be an important factor in relapse to drinking.

Sleep Deprivation And Cardiovascular Problems In Abstinent Alcoholics: Alcohol dependence is a major risk factor for cardiovascular disease, with alcoholic men showing an increased prevalence of hypertension and cardiac arrhythmias. Sleep deprivation induces elevated heart rate and levels of epinephrine and norepinephrine in male alcohol-dependent patients compared to healthy nonalcoholic individuals. These elevations in heart rate and hormone levels do not recover even after a full night of recovery sleep. Abstinent alcoholic individuals show an extended course of sleep problems that can persist for months or years. Therefore, increased nervous system activity that occurs along with habitual sleep loss could play a role in tremor, anxiety, hypertension, and cardiac arrhythmias of abstinent alcoholic subjects.

National Cancer Institute

The National Cancer Institute (NCI) supports a variety of sleep-related research in patients diagnosed with cancer. Sleep disturbances in this population can occur at any point in the cancer trajectory, from diagnosis through survivorship to end of life. Often, the problem occurs in conjunction with other symptoms, most notably pain and fatigue and may be the result of treatment for the disease or for one or more symptoms, such as pain.

Sleep Disturbances Across The Cancer Continuum: The majority of research projects are exploring sleep disturbances as a co-occurring symptom with pain, fatigue, hot flashes, and depression. Patients and their caregivers are often reluctant to communicate their symptoms to clinicians, and a number of studies are underway that are testing interventions to help patients and their caregivers communicate their sleep disturbances to clinicians, as well as assist clinicians in routinely assessing these symptoms. Family and informal caregivers are assuming increasing responsibilities for the care of their loved ones with cancer. NCI is supporting several studies investigating how the burden of caregiving, such as sleep disturbances, is affecting informal caregivers.

Complementary And Alternative Approaches: Currently, NCI is supporting research projects that are testing hypnosis, acupuncture, exercise, meditation, massage, yoga, and healing touch to relieve the primary symptom of insomnia or to relieve co-occurring symptoms, which may, in turn, alleviate sleep disturbances.

Bio-Behavioral Research: There is increasing attention on understanding the underlying biological mechanisms underlying cancer-related and treatment-related symptoms, such as sleep disorders. One example of this is an exploratory study of the role of cytokines in pancreatic cancer patients experiencing depression. Although depression is the primary symptom under investigation, it is well known that other symptoms (sleep disorders, pain, and anxiety) co-exist within this population and an analysis of these symptoms is included in the study.

National Institute Of Child Health And Human Development

The National Institute of Child Health and Human Development (NICHD) supports and promotes sleep research in infants, children, adults, and in animals with early development resembling that of humans. These studies are designed to gain an understanding of the processes that may be involved in the normal development of behavioral state and physiologic control during sleep, as well as those that accompany sudden infant death syndrome (SIDS), learning deficits, and mental retardation, and changes across the lifespan in reproductive health.

Research Highlights: The pathogenic process that leads to SIDS has been under investigation for many years. One major theory is that infants who are vulnerable to SIDS do not respond appropriately during sleep to low oxygen levels and high carbon dioxide levels in the air during sleep. In animal models, these asphyxiating conditions result in a rapid decrease of oxidative metabolism in tissues. This leads to slow heart rate (bradycardia), episodes of prolonged cessation of breathing (apnea), and hypoxic coma.

NICHD supports studies of how the brain controls breathing during sleep, in animal models and in human congenital central hypoventilation syndrome. Patients with congenital central hypoventilation syndrome (CCHS) have a reduced drive to breathe during sleep, a reduced breathing response to elevated carbon dioxide, and impaired autonomic nervous system regulation, such as control of the cardiovascular and respiratory systems. By comparing the biology of CCHS patients with healthy subjects, we learn about the parts of the brain involved in these functions.

Sleeping on the stomach increases the risk for SIDS. Babies are at much higher risk if they sleep on the back and are placed to sleep on the stomach, without the experience of stomach sleeping. It has been proposed that stomach sleep position increases the likelihood that the infant will become face down in the bedding and rebreathe expired air, which is low in oxygen (hypoxia) and rich in carbon dioxide. Researchers examined the protective behaviors of babies who were either experienced in sleeping on their stomachs or inexperienced. The infants were placed to sleep face down in bedding and as a result began breathing in expired air, and all of the infants aroused. If the babies lifted and turned their head, then the carbon dioxide they breathed in dropped more for a longer time than if the just moved their head and nuzzled the bedding. Infants with experience in stomach sleeping had the best protective responses, with more head lifting and turning. In addition, the inexperienced stomach sleepers spent more time with their face down in the bedding. These studies suggest that protective behaviors are learned, and support the theory that some SIDS infants die because they do not acquire the ability to learn protective behaviors. This could be due to a deficit in the nervous system substrate for learning, or to a deficit in the ability to sense carbon dioxide that does not allow them to develop a learned response to elevated carbon dioxide. The latter is consistent with findings by researchers studying brains from SIDS babies, of unique abnormalities in a network of nerve cells that use serotonin as a transmitter and are responsible for sensing carbon dioxide.

Another theory of SIDS is that some babies have a problem with arousal mechanisms during sleep and don't wake up in response to life-threatening stimuli. Sleep has two main components, active sleep or REM and quiet sleep, which is a deep sleep. Scientists have found that infants who sleep on the stomach spend more time in quiet sleep than infants who sleep on their back. Also, babies take longer to wake up to arousing stimuli in the stomach position compared to the back. Researchers extended this finding by showing that even when the babies who sleep on their stomachs are in active sleep, the brain wave activity is slower in frequency that babies who sleep on their backs. The active sleep in stomach sleepers shows more resemblance to quiet sleep. This may explain the increased arousal thresholds observed in babies who sleep in their stomachs.

National Center For Complementary And Alternative Medicine

Many individuals use complementary and alternative medicine (CAM) therapies to treat sleep disorders. For example, it has been estimated that approximately 1.6 million adults (3.1% of all adults who used CAM) used CAM specifically for sleep problems in 2002. These CAM therapies include the use of dietary supplements such as melatonin and valerian; mind/body approaches such as meditation, and therapies that are part of non-western traditional medical systems, such as acupuncture and yoga.

Insomnia: Chronic insomnia is a significant health problem for many individuals, is often difficult to treat, and can last for years. Furthermore,

♣ It's A Fact!!

Because of the wide use of the dietary supplement, melatonin, for sleep disorders, the National Center for Complementary and Alternative Medicine commissioned the Agency for Healthcare Research and Quality (AHRQ) to conduct a systematic review of published research on this subject to determine the strength of scientific evidence supporting the efficacy of melatonin for sleep disorders. This review found that melatonin appears to be safe, but it may not be effective for treating most primary sleep disorders. However, melatonin may be effective in treating delayed sleep phase syndrome. Finally, the report suggests that the mechanism by which melatonin produces sleepiness in humans is still not well understood.

Source: NHLBI, 2004.

conventional therapeutics can produce unwanted side effects. As a result, many individuals have turned to alternative therapies in search of more effective treatments with lesser side effects. The National Center for Complementary and Alternative Medicine (NCCAM) supports a study using yoga as a treatment for insomnia. Although yoga has been recommended for treatment of insomnia by yoga practitioners, its effectiveness has not been scientifically established. The main goal of this ongoing clinical study is to establish whether a regimen of yoga practice will improve sleep onset latency measured by both subjective and objective criteria. In addition, NCCAM funds an ongoing trial on melatonin for insomnia in the elderly. A significant portion of elderly individuals with insomnia have low endogenous levels of melatonin, which is a normally occurring neurohormone as well as a popular dietary supplement sold to treat a variety of sleep disorders. This clinical study will investigate whether dietary supplements of melatonin will relieve insomnia in these individuals.

Another dietary supplement often used for insomnia and other sleep disorders in valerian. Valerian is derived from the root of the plant *Valeriana officinalis* and is commonly sold as a dietary supplement in the United States and Europe. It is often advertised as having hypnotic properties effective in treating sleep disorders. However, insufficient scientific data exists to determine its true effectiveness. NCCAM is currently supporting a study to evaluate its efficacy for insomnia in healthy older adults.

Finally, NCCAM has recently funded a study to investigate whether homeopathic remedies for insomnia are effective. While quite controversial, homeopathy is widely used to treat a variety of conditions in many countries throughout the world, including Great Britain, Germany, France, Belgium, India, and Mexico. A major aim of this study is to determine whether homeopathic treatments for insomnia, compared to placebo, actually have a physiological effect on stages of sleep using polysomnography and sleep electroencephalography.

Sleep Deprivation Related To Other Diseases: Neurodegenerative diseases, such as Parkinson disease and Alzheimer disease, are often accompanied by sleep disturbances due to pain and/or neurological changes related to the progression of the disease. NCCAM currently supports an ongoing clinical study investigating the efficacy and safety of valerian for the treatment of sleep disturbances in Parkinson disease. In addition, NCCAM supports a study on the use of high intensity light therapy for Alzheimer disease patients in nursing homes. This study will investigate whether high intensity lights installed in nursing home common rooms for various periods of time will contribute to a lessening of problems. If results are positive this could provide a low-risk alternative treatment that is relatively inexpensive once the lighting is installed. Finally, NCCAM has recently funded an investigation of the effect of valerian root on sleep disturbances for individuals with rheumatoid arthritis. This clinical study will investigate whether valerian taken an hour before bedtime will improve sleep outcomes.

Basic Science Research: NCCAM supports basic science research aimed at understanding the underlying biological mechanisms of CAM therapeutic modalities including those used to treat sleep disorders. NCCAM continues to encourage and solicit research on interactions between CAM and conventional therapeutics, including but not limited to interactions between dietary supplements and drugs. This would include the interactions between drugs used to treat sleep disorders and dietary supplements such as valerian and melatonin. In addition, NCCAM currently supports a study to investigate whether the active constituents of hops modulate a lipid signaling pathway believed to induce sleep in mammals.

Circadian Biology: NCCAM supports a study investigating the effect of blue light on sleep-wake regulatory cycles in humans. In addition, NCCAM recently funded research to determine the effect of vitamin B_{12} on the human circadian pacemaker.

National Institute On Drug Abuse

The National Institute on Drug Abuse (NIDA) has a primary research goal to understand brain systems affected by psychoactive drugs of abuse. Sleep disturbances both during use of, and following withdrawal from, such drugs among individuals who are addicted strongly suggest the value of sleep studies for the Institute. Indeed, sleep disturbances often outlast other withdrawal symptoms and may be a cause for relapse. NIDA supports sleep studies' focus on the neurobiology associated with sleep, sleep and circadian cycles, and sleep architecture because some of the neural systems involved in the addiction process are also involved in the sleep architecture. In addition, it is important to study how sleepiness on the one hand and insomnia on the other contribute to drug abuse and to relapse following withdrawal.

Because of the overlap in the neural systems involved in sleep and drug abuse, there is reason to hypothesize that sleep disturbances influence efforts to treat drug abuse or conversely, that drug abuse induces sleep disturbances that exacerbate other health problems. Accordingly, it is possible that treatments for sleep disorders may prove effective in the treatment of drug abuse as well. Sleep disturbances are also reported by smokers withdrawing from nicotine. Significantly, treatments for those wishing to quit smoking, bupropion and/or the nicotine patch also cause sleep disturbances.

A major thrust of research is how using drugs of abuse and withdrawing from drugs of abuse affect sleep cycles and sleep efficiency; how cognitive efficiency is affected either by drugs themselves, or loss of sleep because of drugs; and importantly, are the effects on sleep following drug withdrawal part of the cause in cases of relapse? In a study of cocaine abusers residing on an inpatient unit, sleep duration, efficiency, and onset latency worsened across three days of binge use followed by 15 days of abstinence. By contrast, the patients did not report subjective differences in sleep quality. In this study it was concluded that this dissociation between objective and subjective sleep quality may be contributory to relapse. An ongoing, polysomnographic study of sleep quality following abstinence of marijuana abuse is also being carried out where reported sleep disturbances are systematically documented in heavy users. Finally, a study using phosphorous magnetic resonance spectroscopic imaging following sleep deprivation in withdrawing cocaine or heroin abusers seeks to determine metabolic changes in the anterior cerebrum compared to sleep deprivation in non-users. Continuing studies in these areas promise to inform on biological mechanisms underlying drug abuse vulnerability as related to sleep architecture.

National Institute Of Mental Health

Sleep disorders and sleep disruption associated with various mental disorders produce significant distress and impairment, contributing to the burden of mental illness in our society. As a result, the National Institute of

Mental Health (NIMH) supports a rich portfolio of sleep-related research that spans the basic to clinical research continuum and includes research in sleep disturbances of children, adults, and the elderly. Sleep-related research supported by NIMH includes cellular and molecular mechanisms of circadian and sleep-wake systems, effects of sleep on learning and memory, nosology and epidemiology of sleep disorders, the relationship of sleep disruption to mental illness, and development and evaluation of treatments for sleep disorders.

Restricted Sleep Reduces Hippocampal Cell Survival And Neurogenesis: A body of current research indicates that sleep helps consolidate memories by providing a brain state conducive to structural and functional neural changes, or brain plasticity. A recent study shows that the impact of sleep on memory depends upon the type of memory and the brain structures involved. These findings suggest that sleep restriction differentially affects certain memory and performance tasks. The more the hippocampus is activated in learning a task, the more neurogenesis occurs in this region, and the more severe the effects of sleep loss are on neurogenesis and hippocampus-dependent learning. The study results further our understanding of the functions of sleep and highlight the complexity of assessing the effects of sleep deprivation on various types of memory and performance.

✤ It's A Fact!!

Behavioral and physiological studies support the theory that anxiety interferes with rapid eye movement (REM) sleep and that REM sleep is a very favorable state for the consolidation and integration of memories. Despite these findings, however, why and how anxiety and learning are related to sleep remains poorly understood.

Source: NHLBI, 2004.

A Clock Gene Essential For Circadian Rhythms Also Regulates Long-Term Memory: Circadian rhythms are cyclic daily patterns of physiological and behavioral activity critical to a normal sleep-wake cycle. Investigators have identified clock period genes that are essential for establishing circadian rhythm and have determined the importance of CREB (cAMP-responsive element-binding protein) in maintaining the normal expression of these clock

genes. CREB protein synthesis is also critical to long-term memory. Therefore, these researchers hypothesize that long-term memory may be regulated
by the same clock genes that regulate circadian rhythms.

**Differences In PET Scans Of Depressed Patients During Wake And
Non-REM Sleep:** Sleep disturbance is common in depression and is an important risk factor for depression onset and relapse. Depression is also associated with disrupted sleep patterns including alterations in non-rapid eye
movement (NREM) sleep. To better understand the brain functions associated with sleep disturbance in depressed patients, researchers performed re-
gional cerebral glucose metabolism assessments (for example, PET scans) of
depressed and healthy participants during wake and NREM sleep.

Compared to healthy controls, depressed patients showed a smaller decrease in metabolism from wake to NREM sleep in broad regions of the
brain (for example, thalamus and frontal, parietal, and temporal cortex). These
smaller decreases from wake to NREM sleep, however, appeared to be due
primarily to lower metabolism, particularly in prefrontal regions of the brain,
during waking periods in depressed patients. Prefrontal hypometabolism may
be fundamentally altered in depressed patients or may be the result of sleep
disturbance in these patients.

In contrast, depressed patients showed larger decreases in metabolism from
wake to sleep in ventral and posterior brain structures including the left
amygdala, anterior cingulated cortex, cerebellum, parahippocampal cortex, fusi-
form gyrus, and occipital cortex compared to healthy controls. These larger
decreases from wake to NREM sleep, however, appeared to be due primarily
to increased metabolism in these brain areas during waking periods in depressed patients. The hypermetabolism in these regions is consistent with increased arousal that may interfere with sleep onset and maintenance.

The findings from this study offer intriguing possibilities for the complex
relationship at the neurobiological level between depression and sleep disturbance. In the ventral and posterior regions of the brain, depressed patients
show increased activity compared to healthy controls, both during wake and
sleep states, and this hyperarousal may contribute to the sleep disturbance commonly associated with depression. In the prefrontal regions of the brain,

depressed patients show decreased activity compared to healthy controls during waking periods, and sleep deprivation may contribute to the altered prefrontal cortex function consistently observed in depressed patients. Additional neuroimaging research in sleep and related disorders could further elucidate the relationship of sleep disturbance and mental disorders such as depression.

A Longitudinal Study Of Young Children's Sleep Patterns: During the first five years of life, as many as a third of children have some type of sleep disturbance, yet little is known about the nature, course, or possible risk factors for these sleep disturbances. An NIMH-sponsored study assessed sleep behavior, including video observations of sleep, in 68 families of infants over four years. About a third of the infants were classified as "stable non-self-soothers" who were unable at ages six and nine months to calm themselves back to sleep after awakening. These infants were more likely to have sleep onset problems and to be sleeping with a parent at age two. During the first two years of life, 19% of children had sleep difficulties based on stringent classification criteria. Over time, problems with nighttime awakenings diminished, but sleep onset problems persisted.

Approximately half of children at 2 years of age required parental presence to fall asleep. A quarter of the children slept with their parent(s), but only a third of these parents reported this behavior to be a problem. Intermittent sleeping with parents was not associated with sleep problems at later time points, but a subgroup of parents (9%) consistently slept with their children up to age four, which may reflect difficulty having the child sleep independently once sleeping with the parent(s) becomes routine.

This study documents the considerable sleep difficulties among young children and the impact on their families. Additional research is needed to better understand the sleep difficulties of young children and how parents should respond to minimize long-term sleep problems and reduce the impact of these difficulties on the family.

National Institute Of Neurological Disorders And Stroke

The National Institute of Neurological Disorders and Stroke (NINDS) supports basic and clinical research on the neuroscience of sleep, including studies of fundamental mechanisms of sleep, sleep disorders, and associated complications.

Necessity Of Sleep: For most species of mammals, newborns and young spend more of the 24-hour day resting and sleeping than do their elders. Sleep time gradually decreases approaching adulthood. While sleep appears to be essential for life, NINDS supported investigators found some striking exception to this developmental sleep pattern. Unlike terrestrial mammals, baby killer-whales and bottlenose-dolphins as well as their mothers show little or no typical sleep behavior for the first postpartum month, avoiding obstacles and remaining mobile for 24 hours a day. Over the several months after birth, babies and mothers gradually increase the amount of time they spend resting to normal adult levels, but never exceed these levels. These findings indicate either that sleep may not have the developmental and life-sustaining functions attributed to it, or that whales and dolphins somehow accomplish the important functions of sleep without actually sleeping.

Immune System: Studies on the relationship between sleep and the immune system continue to provide fundamental insights into the reason we sleep and the adverse consequences of not sleeping. We feel sleepy when we have a cold and sick when we have not slept enough. Two substances, tumor necrosis factor alpha and interleukin-1 beta, increase their concentration in the brain after neuronal activity. These substances are proinflammatory and promote immune reactions to clear the brain of themselves along with other unwanted molecules. Tumor necrosis factor alpha and interleukin-1 beta have also been shown to regulate sleep. Recent studies supported by

> ♣ **It's A Fact!!**
> Animal and human studies of sleep and learning have demonstrated that training on various tasks increases subsequent rapid eye movement (REM) sleep, followed by improvement in performance on the learned task. Experiments have demonstrated that experimental activation of a certain REM sleep mechanism, the P-wave, enhances the physiological process of memory. On the other hand, REM sleep deprivation after training blocks the expected performance improvement.
>
> Source: NHLBI, 2004.

NINDS indicate that these substances are produced in response to activation of brain cells and can cause sleep-like slowing of brain waves, even when they are administered to small areas of the brain. Tumor necrosis factor alpha and interleukin-1 beta are also involved in neuronal growth and plasticity. Since the intense neuronal activity of wakefulness causes the release of these immune system substances, many researchers think that sleep is initiated by the immune system and that sleep's purpose is to: regulate the growth of connections between brain cells, clear the brain of substances produced during previous wakefulness, and prepare the brain to function properly during subsequent periods of wakefulness.

Circadian Clock: A detailed understanding of circadian timing mechanisms, the body's "clock" on which the sleep-wake cycle depends, is critical for sleep disorders research. Normal functioning of this clock requires a complex interplay of several genes and the neuropeptides these genes produce. Rapid progress understanding the clock has come from studies of the fruit fly in part because it is possible to breed and study large numbers of flies with various genetic make-ups. Two NINDS-funded studies have identified one neuropeptide, pigment dispersing factor, as key in coordinating the circadian clock of the fruit fly. Abnormalities in the gene that produces pigment dispersing factor disrupt the smooth function of the clock and disrupt behavior. Because mammals have a closely related peptide which may have similar functions in the mammalian circadian clock, these findings have implications for insomnia and related sleep problems in humans.

Narcolepsy: Narcolepsy is a disabling sleep disorder affecting about 200,000 Americans. NINDS supported research on narcolepsy has established the importance of the neurotransmitter, hypocretin, in regulating wakefulness and sleep. Losses and defects in neurons that contain hypocretin cause narcolepsy in humans and animals. However, the mechanisms and extent of damage to hypocretin neurons in narcolepsy is not understood. By conducting post-mortem studies, NINDS-funded investigators found that two neuronal regulating molecules which are normally found in the same neurons as hypocretin, were greatly reduced in patients with narcolepsy compared to normal controls. Studies of this kind may lead to new avenues of therapy that target molecules that are found in hypocretin neurons.

National Institute Of Nursing Research

The National Institute of Nursing Research (NINR) supports sleep research in several areas, including sleep disturbances in people with chronic illness, the effects of sleep deprivation on development and function, and how to manage sleep disturbances in a variety of healthcare settings. NINR-funded scientists are studying sleep-related topics such as: designing behavioral interventions to help people improve their sleep habits; studying the effects of sleep/wake cycle disruptions on premature infant development; and investigating the effects of chemotherapy-related sleep disturbances on the quality of life of cancer patients.

Sleep And Pregnant Women: Women often complain of fatigue and difficulty sleeping during pregnancy, especially as they approach delivery. Researchers studied women who slept less than six hours per night or who experienced frequent sleep disturbances during their pregnancy. These women had significantly longer labors and were 3–4 times more likely to have a cesarean delivery than women who slept 7–8 hours a night with fewer disruptions. These results suggest a need for women to get adequate sleep during their pregnancy, and a need for care providers to communicate the benefits of better sleep during pregnancy to their patients.

Colicky Infants: Infants with colic may cry inconsolably for several hours each day, frustrating both parents and health care providers. New theories link colic to the immaturity of the infant's sleep/wake state regulation. In a controlled trial, NINR-funded scientists tested an intervention that used a program of home visits from nurses to help families cope with infant irritability and promote the development of sleep/wake regulation in the infant. Parents were taught over a two-week period to establish routine daily activity

> **♣ It's A Fact!!**
> Often thought to be the result of lifestyle choices, sleep deprivation appears especially common in adolescence. Wake times imposed by school schedules oppose the maturational tendency toward later bedtimes. A recent study suggests that this shift toward later bedtimes may be in part the result of shifting underlying biology rather than behavioral choices.
>
> Source: NHLBI, 2004.

patterns; provide holding, rocking and other soothing contacts; and establish a period of quiet for themselves to promote rest and recovery. Eight weeks after the intervention began, parents reported that crying had fallen from an average of 5–6 hours to less than one hour per day. In the control group, which received standard care, crying was only reduced to 4 hours per day. These results demonstrate that interventions which establish an infant's sleep/wake cycle and educate parents in caring for their colicky infant may help families improve their quality of life.

Bright-Light Treatment Of Alzheimer Disease: Erratic sleep/wake cycles are a major disabling symptom of Alzheimer disease sufferers. Light levels in long-term care facilities are often low and may affect the circadian clock of residents with Alzheimer disease. In a randomized clinical trial, NINR-funded researchers tested the effect of one hour of bright light exposure on the quality of sleep and wakefulness, and rest/activity cycles, of institutionalized Alzheimer patients. Bright light exposure significantly improved rest/activity rhythms in these patients, but had no effect on quality of nighttime sleep or daytime wakefulness. This study suggests that timed bright light exposure may help to adjust the circadian rhythms of Alzheimer patients to a normal 24-hour day.

Hemodialysis Patients: The majority of patients with end-stage renal disease undergoing hemodialysis (HD) have problems with sleep that affect their quality of life. Sleep/wake cycles are influenced by body temperature (BT), with relatively low BTs occurring prior to the onset of sleep. HD often causes slight elevations in a patient's BT. Because of these two factors, NINR-funded scientists are currently testing the effects of using cool dialysate during HD instead of the warm dialysate normally used in an effort to lower BT and promote sleep. Dialysate is the cleansing solution composed of salts and glucose used during dialysis. Researchers will monitor the sleep/wake cycles of patients receiving the intervention, as well as patients' behavioral and physiological functioning. Findings from this research may assist care providers in improving the quality of life of patients undergoing HD.

Improving Sleep In Persons With Dementia: Persons with cognitive disorders often suffer from sleep disturbances, especially those in long-term care facilities. Drug treatments often prove ineffective at combating these

♣ **It's A Fact!!**
Sleep Disturbance In The Chronically Ill

Sleep disturbances significantly contribute to the burden of illness in many chronic health conditions. In addition to the effects of pain disturbing sleep, changes in physiologic processes may interfere with normal sleep patterns. For example, Alzheimer disease, dementia, rheumatoid arthritis, fibromyalgia, AIDS, asthma, and urinary incontinence are all accompanied by sleep disruptions.

Source: NHLBI, 2004.

sleep problems. In a randomized controlled trial, NINR-funded scientists are testing a behavioral intervention for its ability to improve the sleep quality of nursing home residents. The treatment will involve social activities such as listening to music or playing games, progressive resistance training of the hips and arms, or both. A control group will receive usual treatment. Sleep and wake quality will be measured after seven weeks. This intervention may inform clinicians of the usefulness of innovative behavioral interventions in improving the sleep quality and quality of life of patients with dementia.

Recovery Of Neurobehavioral Functioning: Chronic sleep loss due to medical conditions or other factors is known to affect normal daily functioning and cause health problems. NINR-funded researchers are currently determining the amount and types of sleep necessary to recover normal behavioral and physiological function following sleep deprivation. These scientists are testing a group of healthy subjects who have been kept awake and then allowed to sleep, both for varying amounts of time. The investigators are monitoring behavioral and physiological functioning while the subjects are awake and are measuring physiological states while the subjects are asleep. Findings from this research could lead to an improved theoretical understanding of the relationship between sleep and neurobehavioral function, and lead to the development of better interventions and guidelines for the public regarding sleep and health.

Part Six

If You Need More Information

Chapter 45

Resources For Additional Information About Sleep And Sleep Disorders

American Academy of Neurology
1080 Montreal Avenue
Saint Paul, MN 55116
Toll-Free: 800-879-1960
Phone: 651-695-2717
Fax: 651-695-2791
Website: http://www.aan.com
E-mail: memberservices@aan.com

American Academy of Otolaryngology/Head and Neck Surgery
One Prince Street
Alexandria, VA 22314-3357
Phone: 703-836-4444
Fax: 703-683-5100
TTY: 703-519-1585
Website: http://www.entnet.org
E-mail: info@entnet.org

American Academy of Sleep Medicine
One Westbrook Corporate Center
Suite 920
Westchester, IL 60154
Phone: 708-492-0930
Fax: 708-492-0943
Website: http://www.aasmnet.org

American Board of Sleep Medicine
One Westbrook Corporate Center
Suite 920
Westchester, IL 60154
Phone: 708-492-1290
Fax: 708-492-0943
Website: http://www.absm.org
E-mail: absm@absm.org

American Chronic Pain Association

P.O. Box 850
Rocklin, CA 95677
Toll-Free: 800-533-3231
Phone: 916-632-0922
Fax: 916-632-3208
Website: http://www.theacpa.org
E-mail: ACPA@pacbell.net

American College of Chest Physicians

3300 Dundee Road
Northbrook, IL 60062-2348
Toll-Free: 800-343-2227
Phone: 847-498-1400
Website: http://www.chestnet.org

American Insomnia Association

One Westbrook Corporate Center
Suite 920
Westchester, IL 60154
Phone: 708-492-0930
Fax: 708-492-0943
Website: http://www.american
insomniaassociation.org
E-mail: aiainfo@aasmnet.org

American Psychiatric Association

1000 Wilson Boulevard, Suite 1825
Arlington, VA 22209-3901
Toll-Free: 888-35-PSYCH
(888-357-7924)
Phone: 703-907-7300
Fax: 703-907-1085
Website: http://www.psych.org
E-mail: apa@psych.org

American Psychological Association

750 First Street, NE
Washington, DC 20002-4242
Toll-Free: 800-374-2721
Phone: 202-336-5500
TDD/TTY: 202-336-6123
Website: http://www.apa.org

American Sleep Apnea Association

1424 K Street NW, Suite 302
Washington, DC 20005
Phone: (202) 293-3650
Fax: (202) 293-3656
Website: http://www.sleepapnea.org
E-mail: asaa@sleepapnea.org

American Association of Sleep Technology

One Westbrook Corporate Center
Suite 920
Westchester, IL 60154
Website: http://www.asstweb.org

Better Sleep Council

501 Wythe Street
Alexandria, VA 22314-1917
Website: http://
www.bettersleep.org
E-mail: bsc@sleepproducts.org

Center for Sleep Research, UCLA

Website: http://www.npi.ucla.edu/
sleepresearch

International Association for the Study of Dreams

1672 University Avenue
Berkeley, CA 94703
Phone: 209-724-0889
Website: http://www.asdreams.org
E-mail: office@asdreams.org

Kidzzzsleep

Rhode Island Hospital
593 Eddy Street
Providence, RI 02903
http://www.kidzzzsleep.org

Klein-Levin Syndrome Foundation

P.O. Box 5382
San Jose, CA 95150-5382
Phone 408-265-1099
Fax: 408-269-2131
Website: http://
www.klsfoundation.org
E-mail: facts@klsfoundation.org

Narcolepsy Network, Inc.

79A Main Street
North Kingstown, RI 02852
Toll-Free: 888-292-6522
Phone: 401-667-2523
Fax 401-633-6567
Website: http://
www.narcolepsynetwork.org
E-mail:
narnet@narcolepsynetwork.org

National Center for Complementary and Alternative Medicine

P.O. Box 7923
Gaithersburg, MD 20898
Toll-Free: 888-644-6226
Phone: 301-519-3153
TTY: 866-464-3615
Fax: 866-464-3616
Website: http://nccam.nih.gov
E-mail: info@nccam.nih.gov

National Center on Sleep Disorders Research
National Heart, Lung, and Blood Institute
Health Information Center
P.O. Box 30105
Bethesda, MD 20824-0105
Phone: 301-592-8573
TTY: 240-629-3255
Fax: 301-592-8563
Website: http://www.nhlbi.nih.gov/about/ncsdr
E-mail: nhlbiinfo@nhlbi.nih.gov

National Highway Traffic Safety Administration
1200 New Jersey Avenue, SE
West Building
Washington, DC 20590
Toll-Free: 888-DASH-2-DOT
(888-327-4236)
Website: http://www.nhtsa.dot.gov
E-mail: webmaster@nhtsa.dot.gov

National Institute of Child Health and Human Development
31 Center Drive
Bethesda, MD 20892-2425
Phone: 800-370-2943
Fax: 301-496-7101
Website: http://www.nichd.nih.gov
E-mail:
NICHDInformationResourceCenter
@mail.nih.gov

National Institute of Neurological Disorders and Stroke
P.O. Box 5801
Bethesda, MD 20824
Toll-Free: 800-352-9424
Phone: 301-496-5751
TTY: 301-468-5981
Website: http://www.ninds.nih.gov

National Institute on Mental Health
6001 Executive Boulevard
Room 8184, MSC 9663
Bethesda, MD 20892-9663
Toll Free: 866-615-NIMH (6464)
Phone: 301-443-4513
TTY: 866-415-8051
Fax: 301-443-4279
Website: http://www.nimh.nih.gov
E-mail: nimhinfo@nih.gov

National Sleep Foundation
1522 K Street, NW, Suite 500
Washington, DC 20005
Phone: 202-347-3471
Fax: 202-347-3472
Website: http://
www.sleepfoundation.org
E-mail: nsf@sleepfoundation.org

Nemours Foundation Center for Children's Health Media

1600 Rockland Road
Wilmington, DE 19803
Phone: 302-651-4000
Website: http://www.kidshealth.org
E-mail: info@kidshealth.org

Restless Legs Syndrome Foundation

1610 14th St. NW, Suite 300
Rochester, MN 55901
Toll-Free: 877-463-6757
Phone: 507-287-6465
Fax: 507-287-6312
Website: http://www.rls.org
E-mail: rlsfoundation@rls.org

Sleep and Health

Website: http://
www.sleepandhealth.com
E-mail: office@sleepandhealth.com

Sleep Research Society

One Westbrook Corporate Center
Suite 920
Westchester, IL 60154
Website: http://
www.sleepresearchsociety.org

SleepNet.com

http://www.sleepnet.com

Society for Light Treatment and Biological Rhythms

4648 Main Street
Chincoteague, VA 23336
Fax: 757-336-5777
http://www.websciences.org/sltbr
E-mail: sltbrinfo@aol.com

Society for Neuroscience

1121 14th St. NW, Suite 1010
Washington DC 20005
Phone: 202-462-6688
Fax: 202-962-4941
Website: http://web.sfn.org
E-mail: info@sfn.org

Society for Research on Biological Rhythms

University of Illinois at Urbana-
Champaign
302 East John St., Suite 202
Champaign, IL 61820
Phone: 217-333-2880
Fax: 217-333-9561
Website: http://www.srbr.org

Stanford University Center for Narcolepsy

Department of Psychiatry and
Behavioral Sciences
1201 Welch Road, Room P112
Stanford, CA 94305-5485
Fax: 650-725-4913
Website: http://www-
med.stanford.edu/school/
Psychiatry/narcolepsy/index.html

Stanford University Center of Excellence for the Diagnosis and Treatment of Sleep Disorders

Website: http://www.med.stanford
.edu/school/psychiatry/coe

Star Sleeper Campaign

National Heart, Lung, and Blood
Institute
Website: http://www.nhlbi.nih.gov/
health/public/sleep/starslp

Sudden Infant Death Syndrome Alliance/First Candle

1314 Bedford Avenue, Suite 210
Baltimore, MD 21208
Toll-Free: 800-221-7437
Website: http://
www.sidsalliance.org
E-mail: info@firstcandle.org

Talk About Sleep, Inc.

14480 Ewing Ave So., Suite 102
Burnsville, MN 55306
Website: http://
www.talkaboutsleep.com
E-mail: info@talkaboutsleep.com

The Sleep Site

1430 South High Street
Columbus, OH 43207
Phone: 614-443-7800
Fax: 614-443-6960
Website: http://
www.thesleepsite.com

U.S. Consumer Product Safety Commission

Washington, DC 20207-0001
Phone: 800-638-2772
TTY: 800-638-8270
Fax: 301-504-0124
Website: http://www.cpsc.gov
E-mail: info@cpsc.gov

WetBusters.com: A Bedwetting Site for Kids and Teens

2800 Elliott Ave, Suite 1430
Seattle, WA 98121
Phone: 206-448-4414
Website: http://www.wetbuster.com
E-mail: feedback@wetbusters.com

World Federation of Sleep Research Societies

http://www.wfsrs.org

Chapter 46

Suggestions For Further Reading About Sleep And Sleep Disorders

Books about Sleep and Sleep Disorders

To make topics easier to identify, books in this section are listed alphabetically by title.

Coping with Sleep Disorders
by Carolyn Simpson; Publisher: Rosen Publishing Group, 1996
ISBN: 9780823920686

Dead on Their Feet: The Health Effects of Sleep Deprivation in Teens
by Joan Esherick; Publisher: Mason Crest Publishers, 2004
ISBN: 9781590848456

Getting a Good Night's Sleep
by Nancy Foldvary-Schaefer; Publisher: Cleveland Clinic Press, 2006
ISBN: 9781596240148

Good Night: The Sleep Doctor's 4-Week Program to Better Sleep and Better Health
by Michael Breus; Publisher: Penguin Group (USA), 2006
ISBN: 9780525949794

Harvard Medical School Guide to a Good Night's Sleep
by Lawrence J. Epstein with Steven Mardon; Publisher: McGraw-Hill, 2006
ISBN: 9780071467438

100 Questions and Answers about Sleep and Sleep Disorders
by Sudhansu Chokroverty; Publisher: Blackwell Publishers, 2001
ISBN: 9780865425835

101 Questions about Sleep and Dreams That Kept You Awake Nights...until Now
by Faith Hickman Brynie; Publisher: Twenty-First Century Books, 2006
ISBN: 9780761323129

Promise of Sleep: A Pioneer in Sleep Medicine Explores the Vital Connection between Health, Happiness, and a Good Night's Sleep
by William C. Dement with Christopher Vaughan; Publisher: Dell Publishing, 1999
ISBN: 9780440509011

Restless Legs Syndrome: Relief and Hope for Sleepless Victims of a Hidden Epidemic
by Robert H. Yoakum; Publisher: Simon and Schuster, 2006
ISBN: 9780743280686

Sleep: The Mysteries, the Problems, and the Solutions
by Carlos H. Schenck; Publisher: Penguin Group (USA), 2007
ISBN: 9781583332702

Sleep Disorders
by Gail B. Stewart; Publisher: Thomson Gale, 2002
ISBN: 9781560069096

Sleep Disorders For Dummies
by Max Hirshkowitz, William C. Dement, Patricia B. Smith; Publisher:
Wiley, John and Sons, Inc., 2004
ISBN: 9780764539015

Sleep Disorders Sourcebook: Basic Consumer Health Information about Sleep and Sleep Disorders, Including Insomnia, Sleep Apnea, Restless Legs Syndrome, Narcolepsy, Parasomnias, and Other Health Problems That Affect Sleep, Plus Facts about Diagnostic Procedures, Treatment Strategies, Sleep Medications, and Tips for Improving Sleep Quality; Along with a Glossary of Related Terms and Resources for Additional Help and Information
by Amy L. Sutton; Publisher: Omnigraphics, 2005
ISBN: 9780780807433

Sleeping Well: The Sourcebook for Sleep and Sleep Disorders
by Jan Yager and Michael J. Thorpy; Publisher: Facts on File, 2001
ISBN: 9780816040902

Sleepless in America: Is Your Child Misbehaving or Missing Sleep?
by Mary Sheedy Kurcinka; Publisher: HarperCollins Publishers, 2007
ISBN: 9780060736026

Snooze or Lose: 10 "No-War" Ways to Improve Your Teen's Sleep Habits
by Helene A. Emsellem with Carol Whiteley; Publisher: National
Academies Press, 2006
ISBN: 9780309101899

Take Charge of Your Child's Sleep: The All-in-One Resource for Solving Sleep Problems in Kids and Teens
by Judith A. Owens and Jodi Mindell; Publisher: Avalon Publishing
Group, 2005
ISBN: 9781569243626

Understanding Sleep and Dreaming
by William H. Moorcroft; Publisher: Springer-Verlag, 2005
ISBN: 9780306474255

Web-Based Resources

Healthfinder.gov
http://www.healthfinder.gov
Click on "Sleep" and "Sleep Disorders"

How Sleep Works
How Stuff Works
http://health.howstuffworks.com/sleep.htm

How to Get Great Sleep
Psychology Today
http://psychologytoday.com/articles/pto-3097.html

Sleep
Nova Science Now (PBS)
http://www.pbs.org/wgbh/nova/sciencenow/3410/01.html

Sleep Apnea
MedlinePlus
http://www.nlm.nih.gov/medlineplus/sleepapnea.html

Sleep Center
Mayo Clinic
http://www.mayoclinic.com/health/sleep/SL99999

Sleep Disorders
MedlinePlus
http://www.nlm.nih.gov/medlineplus/sleepdisorders.html

Sleep Disorders Health Center
WebMD
http://www.webmd.com/sleep-disorders

Sleep for Kids
A Service of the National Sleep Foundation
http://www.sleepforkids.org

SleepChannel
Healthcommunities.com
http://www.sleepdisorderchannel.com

Star Sleeper for Kids
National Heart, Lung, and Blood Institute
http://www.nhlbi.nih.gov/health/public/sleep/starslp/index.htm

Topic: Sleep
American Psychological Association (APA) Online
http://www.apa.org/topics/topicsleep.html

What Is Sleep and Why We Do It
Neuroscience for Kids
http://faculty.washington.edu/chudler/sleep.html

Your Guide to Healthy Sleep
MedicineNet
http://www.medicinenet.com/sleep/article.htm

U.S. Racking Up Huge Sleep Debt
National Geographic News
http://news.nationalgeographic.com/news/2005/02/
0224_050224_sleep.html

Index

Index

Page numbers that appear in *Italics* refer to illustrations. Page numbers that have a small 'n' after the page number refer to information shown as Notes at the beginning of each chapter. Page numbers that appear in **Bold** refer to information contained in boxes on that page (except Notes information at the beginning of each chapter).